Sexuality

AFTER CANCER TREATMENT

Judy C. Kneece, RN, OCN

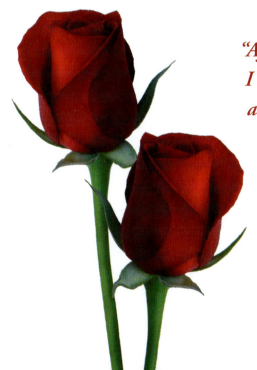

*"After cancer treatment,
I want my life back ...
and that includes my sex life."*

— Anonymous Patient

Copyright © 2017 Judy C. Kneece, RN, OCN

2017: 1st Edition, 1st Printing

All rights reserved. Reproduction or use of editorial or pictorial content in any manner is prohibited without written permission, except in the case of brief quotations embodied in articles or reviews. Readers accessing an on-line version of this work in an authorized manner are permitted to download or print one copy for personal viewing. Other reproduction, distribution or use of copyrightable content without the express written consent of the copyright owner is prohibited. Permission can be requested by contacting the author at: 8420 Dorchester Road, Suite 203, North Charleston, SC 29420.

No patent liability is assumed with respect to the use of the information contained herein. While every precaution has been taken in the preparation of this book, the publisher and author assume no responsibility for errors or omissions. Neither is any liability assumed for damages resulting from the use of the information contained herein. This book has been written to enlighten women and motivate them to discuss the issues with their healthcare team. Patients should determine the best treatment protocol based on physicians' recommendations and their own needs, assessments and desires.

All trademarks used in this book are the property of their respective owners.

ISBN: 978-1-886665-35-4

Library of Congress Control Number: 2017935246

Printed in the United States of America

Published by EduCare Publishing Inc.

To Order:
 EduCare Publishing Inc.
 8420 Dorchester Road, Suite 203
 North Charleston, SC 29420
 1-800-849-9271 or Fax: 843-760-6988
 www.educareinc.com

Illustrations: Alila Medical Media, Debra Strange, Jeremy Darby

About the Author

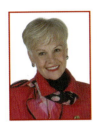

Judy C. Kneece, RN, OCN, is a certified oncology nurse with a specialty in breast cancer. She began her career in 1991 as a Breast Health Navigator, where she developed her concept of patient navigation. In 1994, she started EduCare Inc. to train other nurses as Breast Health Navigators and to write educational information for breast cancer patients.

During the past twenty-three years, EduCare Inc. has been a leader in developing educational materials and in training nurses to support breast cancer patients. Judy has trained over 2,300 nurses to fill the Breast Health Navigator role in hospitals, breast centers and physicians' offices.

Judy is the author of the following breast health books: *Breast Cancer Treatment Handbook, Breast Cancer Support Partner Handbook, Breast Cancer Survivorship Handbook, Solving the Mystery of Breast Pain, Solving the Mystery of Breast Discharge* and the *Breast Health Navigator Manual*. She also created the *COPE Library: Breast Health Edition*, a collection of over 450 patient education topics.

Her background as a Breast Health Navigator has allowed her to witness the struggles cancer survivors have in the area of sexuality following cancer treatment. While most side effects of cancer treatment have an abundance of patient education available, sexuality side effects have often been overlooked or ignored. It was through her experiences with patients that she recognized the need women have for information about restoring their sexual functioning. She realized the importance of putting information in the hands of women seeking help. This book is written to help women identify their individual challenges and inform them of options available to help alleviate or eliminate sexual side effects.

Judy currently serves as a national consultant for breast centers and hospitals. She serves as a member of the American College of Surgeons' Education Committee for the National Accreditation Program for Breast Centers (NAPBC) and on the advisory board for the Clinical Breast Care Project. She has served as a contributing editor for numerous national women's magazines on the issues of breast health and cancer and has over 40 nationally published articles on breast care topics. Judy speaks widely to patients on triumphant survivorship.

Dedication

This book is dedicated to all of the patients, Breast Health Navigators and breast centers who participated in one of the eleven EduCare *Sexuality After Breast Cancer Treatment* focus groups held in 2000 and 2001.

I would like to thank the following breast cancer centers that opened up their facilities and provided staff for hosting the focus groups. Without their cooperation, it would have been impossible to gain a clear, concise understanding of the impact of chemotherapy on a patient's sex life.

Elliott Hospital, Manchester, New Hampshire
Kettering Medical Center, Dayton, Ohio
Grant Riverside Methodist Hospital, Columbus, Ohio
St. Francis Hospital, Indianapolis, Indiana
Southern Illinois University, Springfield, Illinois
Don and Sybil Harrington Cancer Center, Amarillo, Texas
Scripps, San Diego, California
Northside Hospital, Atlanta, Georgia
St. Joseph's Women's Hospital, Tampa, Florida
Lexington Medical Center, Columbia, South Carolina
Breast Cancer Support Groups, Diana Wall, Las Vegas, Nevada

An even greater appreciation goes to each of the breast cancer patients who attended one of these eleven focus groups. These courageous women generously gave three hours of their time to share about the impact breast cancer treatment had on their sexual lives. They did this to help other women who would one day share their same experience. Their honest answers to intimate questions provided the information needed to compile a summary of sexual problems that are common to women after cancer treatment. From this summary, thousands of breast cancer patients have benefited by knowing what to expect and understanding that this is a common struggle.

To these 126 focus group participants, I will be forever grateful for their time, their openness and their participation. These women forged a path to understanding sexuality after cancer treatment. Their willingness to share will continue to benefit other patients who will be following the same path of a cancer diagnosis and treatment for years to come.

Dear Cancer Survivor

Congratulations! If you are reading this book, it means you were diagnosed, treated and have survived cancer. Welcome to one of your final survivorship challenges—restoring your normal sex life.

When you were diagnosed with cancer, you had only one sensible choice, and that was to seek help to rid your body of something potentially life-threatening. The good news was there were proven treatments for your cancer. Today, the not-so-good news is that after receiving treatment you may be left dealing with lingering side effects caused by your life-saving cancer treatment. These side effects are not only bothersome, but they may also interfere with your sex life. However, the side effects of treatment serve as a reminder that your cancer was treatable. Because of cancer treatment, you had the opportunity to confront a life-threatening disease and to become a survivor of cancer instead of a statistic.

Since your diagnosis, you have, no doubt, faced and overcome many challenges to arrive at a place in your journey where you can now turn your interest from fighting cancer to thriving as a cancer survivor. During treatment, sexual functioning issues were probably very low priority on your list of problems to be solved. Now that cancer treatment is behind you, it is time to address any residual side effects on your sexuality.

As a cancer survivor, the question becomes, *"What can I do to restore my sexual functioning?"* That is the purpose of this book—to serve as a guide to help you understand what you can do. In this book, we will discuss the potential side effects you may be encountering that keep you from having the sex life you once had. We will also share ways that you can manage, minimize or eliminate the side effects. And, if you did not find sex enjoyable before treatment, maybe you will find some new interventions and advice to "spice up" your sex life. Together, you and your sexual partner can find enjoyment in your sexual relationship once again.

It is my privilege to be your guide on this journey toward experiencing full survivorship. Let's get started on your sexual restoration!

Your partner in sexual recovery,

Judy

Table of Contents

Copyright ii
About the Author iii
Dedication iv
Dear Cancer Survivor v
Table of Contents vi
Getting the Most Out of This Book viii

Chapter Titles

Chapter 1	Sexuality After Cancer Treatment	1
Chapter 2	Factors Affecting Sex Drive	11
	Personal Quality of Life Pre-Assessment	18
Chapter 3	Female Sexual Anatomy	21
Chapter 4	Effect of Hormones on Sexuality	31
Chapter 5	Vaginal Dryness and Painful Intercourse	43
Chapter 6	Urinary Changes	59
Chapter 7	Hot Flashes and Night Sweats	65
Chapter 8	Fatigue	71
Chapter 9	Sleep Problems	75
Chapter 10	Depression and Anxiety	81
Chapter 11	Value of Exercise	93
Chapter 12	Value of Nutrition	101
Chapter 13	The Single Woman and Future Sexual Intimacy	111
Chapter 14	Drugs That Lower Your Sex Drive	115
Chapter 15	Understanding Female Sex Drive	123
Chapter 16	Increasing Female Sexual Pleasure	135

Chapter 17	Desire-Enhancing Medications and Supplements	153
Chapter 18	Reclaiming Your Life After Cancer	161
	Personal Quality of Life Post-Assessment	166
A Final Word		169

Appendix and Reference

Appendix A	Comparison of Breast Reconstruction Procedures	173
Appendix B	Vaginal Dilator Therapy	179
Appendix C	Sexuality After Breast Cancer Treatment Focus Group Study	181
Bibliography		189
Index		191

Tear-Out Supplement

A Message to the Sexual Partner	197

Getting the Most Out of This Book

This book was written to lead you, step-by-step, in understanding the potential causes of your sexual dysfunction. Because each person has unique circumstances and a wide range of contributing factors, each chapter carefully explains possible causes and what can be done to decrease or alleviate identified problems. As you read through this book, you will gain the information needed to help your sex life come alive again.

I highly suggest that you read the chapters in the order they are presented to evaluate every possible contributing cause. However, I know some women may want to "skip ahead" to the section about what happens in the bedroom. This information begins in *Chapter 15: Understanding Female Sex Drive*.

Good sex is like a good recipe. If you leave out any ingredient, you will not get the outcome you want. Be sure you read all of the chapters so you will not miss an essential ingredient in your quest to restore your sex life.

Bonus: **A Message to The Sexual Partner**

Your sexual partner plays a pivotal role in your sexual healing. With their understanding and support, your sexual restoration becomes much easier. When I was conducting the national *Sexuality After Breast Cancer Treatment* focus groups, I asked the participants if they felt comfortable sharing the details of how cancer treatment had changed their sexual functioning with their partner or if they preferred someone else tell them. To my surprise, 90 percent of the participants responded that they did not feel comfortable and preferred someone else explain what had happened to their body during treatment.

To help you with this much-needed conversation, I have included a brief explanation for your partner. It explains the sexuality changes caused by chemotherapy and how your partner can help you in your quest for sexual restoration. The information is provided on tear-out sheets so you can remove them from the book and give them to your partner. The tear-out supplement begins on page 197.

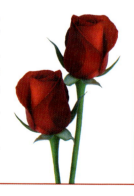

Chapter 1

Sexuality After Cancer Treatment

It is estimated that 850,000 females are diagnosed with cancer each year. The majority of these women undergo chemotherapy to eradicate cancer from their body. The good news is that chemotherapy has increased cancer survival rates to an all-time high. The not-so-good news is that approximately 70 percent of these women are left with unexpected changes in their sex life—changes that are not life-threatening but disrupt the quality of their life. After treatment, they experience an extreme drop in their level of desire, find arousal difficult, experience a lack of lubrication during arousal and find the former pleasure of orgasm elusive. Along with these changes, they also experience hot flashes, night sweats, insomnia, urinary changes, weight changes, mood changes, fatigue and a number of other problems.

These sexuality changes usually come as a complete surprise to patients because they were not forewarned by their healthcare provider. Naturally, patients expect changes during treatment, but they don't realize that many side effects will linger long after treatment is over and, especially, that they will continue to affect their sex life.

Because these changes are not life-threatening, they often go unaddressed unless a patient returns to her healthcare provider for specific help. Instead, many women suffer in silence, attributing their problems to personal inadequacies. Patients often think that this is the price they have to pay for being cancer-free.

Suffering in silence is over. This book will explore the sexuality problems you may be facing and will provide interventions to help reduce or eliminate these side effects.

Chapter 1

The Common Struggle

If you are experiencing changes in your sex life, you should understand that many women share this common struggle after cancer treatment. The *Journal of Sexual Medicine*, reported in the article, *"Sexual Function After Breast Cancer,"* the findings of a study involving 994 cancer-treated female patients. All the patients surveyed were sexually active and had a sexual partner at the time of diagnosis. Two years after cancer treatment ended, 70 percent of these patients, under 70 years of age, reported they were still experiencing sexual difficulties.

Even though the percentage of patients affected by lingering sexual problems is very high, it is one of the least-discussed side effects after cancer treatment. Cancer survivors are often left on their own to find ways to deal with the side effects and regain their pre-cancer sexual functioning.

Patient Focus Groups to Identify Sexuality Issues

As a nurse working directly with patients, I witnessed the struggles survivors had in learning what they could do to return to their previous level of sexual functioning. I listened to their stories about loss of sexual desire and painful sex. I also heard about the lack of help they received from their physicians in dealing with their problems. No one seemed to clearly understand what sexuality side effects chemo-treated patients were dealing with or what could be done to help.

In 2000, I was updating my patient-sexuality lecture for a training I was conducting for nurses. My goal for the patient-sexuality lecture was to provide nurses with practical information they could share with patients to help them deal with sexuality problems encountered after chemotherapy. While researching medical journals to prepare for the lecture, I found that the available literature provided little insight into the problems patients experienced. I wanted to understand more about the experiences of women who had undergone chemotherapy and how it affected their sexual functioning and quality of life.

To fill this information gap, I conducted eleven national *Sexuality After Breast Cancer Treatment* focus groups with breast cancer patients who had received chemotherapy. The focus groups investigated the physical and sexual changes experienced, the impact of changes in the relationship

Sexuality After Cancer Treatment

with the sexual partner, the education received before treatment and requests for future services in education and support.

A total of 126 survivors attended the focus groups and each one responded to 143 questions using individual audience response pads. These handheld computer pads allowed all answers to be anonymous. Each woman was free to express her true feelings. A computer program analyzed the data entered at each site and then combined the data from the eleven sites for the final analysis. A list of the participating facilities and the process of data collection is included in *Appendix C* at the end of this book.

Throughout this book, you will find the combined focus group responses to help you understand what other women have experienced after cancer treatment. Data from the groups is presented as an average percentage (0% – 100%) or an average of a self-evaluation scale (1 – 10).

The summary of the focus group participants' lingering side effects experienced one year after treatment completion is provided below.

Patient Side Effects Experienced One Year After Chemotherapy Treatment

Side Effect of Treatment	Percentage of Change From Time of Diagnosis to One Year After Treatment	
Orgasm Ability	47%	Decrease
Sex Drive	42%	Decrease
Self Body Image	24%	Decrease
Energy	22%	Decrease
Painful Intercourse	163%	Increase
Vaginal Dryness	158%	Increase
Hot Flashes	83%	Increase
Depression	75%	Increase
Night Sweats	65%	Increase
Insomnia	61%	Increase
Anxiety	33%	Increase
Mood Swings	22%	Increase
Anger / Aggression	12%	Increase
Weight Gain	54%	Gained

— *EduCare Focus Group Data*

Chapter 1

> **Change in Sexual Functioning**
> - 14% reported no change in frequency of sex
> - 4% reported increased frequency of sex
> - 82% reported decreased frequency of sex
>
> — *EduCare Focus Group*

Sexuality Focus Group Findings

Conducting the focus groups provided me with insight into what chemo-treated patients had to deal with as they were rebuilding their lives after cancer treatment. Unaddressed side effects of treatment had lowered their overall quality of life. The impact of chemotherapy had greatly altered their sex lives. As we continue through this book, each side effect listed in the chart above will be addressed, along with suggestions to help you reduce, alter or eliminate the side effect.

Common Patient Experiences

When the survey data was compiled, the common identified needs of the patients provided an understanding about what had happened to them. Most of them agreed that they did not regret their decision to have chemotherapy because it was the treatment component that eradicated their cancer. However, they simply wanted to know what they could do now to restore their sexual functioning.

Lack of Patient Education About Potential Sexual Problems

One of the most surprising issues we identified during our national focus groups was that patients had not been forewarned of possible sexual changes after treatment. EduCare's *Sexuality After Breast Cancer Treatment* focus group data revealed that only 13 percent of patients had a discussion

> **Sex Drive**
>
> *"Is this not a case for medical malpractice? Giving us drugs that cause problems that they never mention before they give them?"*
>
> — *Patient, EduCare Focus Group*

with a healthcare provider before treatment began that warned them of the potential changes in their sexual functioning after cancer treatment. An additional 5 percent of patients surveyed had a sexuality discussion with a healthcare provider after treatment began. This resulted in a total of only 18 percent of the 127 patients ever having a sexuality discussion with a healthcare provider. The overwhelming majority of chemotherapy-treated patients, 82 percent, were **not** forewarned of any changes in their sexual functioning.

Sexuality Education

In 2009, the Association of Reproductive Health Professionals conducted a survey of 304 healthcare professionals. The survey focused on patients' discussion of sexuality issues during physician appointments. The survey revealed:

- 50% of interviewed healthcare professionals reported sexual health was the least commonly discussed topic with female patients.
- 39% of interviewed healthcare professionals reported discussing sexual problems with their patients.
- 74% of the healthcare professionals that discussed sexual problems reported that they depended on the patient to initiate the discussion.

It is evident from this survey that many healthcare professionals who practice in the area of cancer treatment may not address sexual issues. If you have not gotten answers to your questions or guidance on how to deal with side effects impacting your sexual function, that is the purpose of this book.

Misplaced Patient Blame

During the focus groups, I also discovered that many of the women wrongly blamed themselves for their sexual problems. When the attendees learned that their lack of sex drive was **not** something they were personally responsible for, but was a side effect of the drugs they were given to treat their cancer, a sense of relief filled the room. As I explained this to one focus group, I vividly remember a young woman bursting into tears and telling me she wished her husband could hear this information. She continued to share that she had been struggling for two years under the weight of not being able to regain normal sexual functioning and had blamed herself for the inability to return to normal.

I also discovered that, because of their decreased sex drive, some women were blamed by their sexual partner for "not being interested in them" or "not being in love with them anymore." This type of personal accusation had resulted in severe emotional pain, often for years, for many of the focus group participants. Accusations that blame the patient for their

Chapter 1

reduced sex drive are an emotional burden that no cancer patient should ever have to endure.

> **Partners' Interpretation of Sexual Changes**
>
> *"Did your partner interpret the changes in your sex drive to a lack of personal interest or desire for the relationship?"*
> - 22% reported that their partners felt they had lost interest in them
> - 22% reported that they did not know what their partners thought
> - 56% reported that their partners did not interpret the change as such
>
> — *EduCare Focus Group*

Low sex drive is an expected side effect of most chemotherapy treatments. Sadly, this information is often neglected in health care discussions with patients, much less shared with the patient's sexual partner. Instead, women are left to struggle alone, trying to make sense of what is happening and searching for answers.

Personal Experience of One Patient

In one of our sexuality focus groups, I received a hand-written note detailing one patient's experience with sexuality changes after chemotherapy. Her experience expresses the challenges many cancer patients face:

> *"My husband was very loving during treatment; he hugged and complimented me lots and often he would just reach out to touch me to let me know he was there. Because I was so violently ill during treatment (I had treatment before Zofran), he never approached me for intercourse. However, after treatment, he felt very rejected because I had no desire for sex and was unable to respond to him sexually. This caused a lot of stress and negative feelings for three years.*
>
> *I had been reading and asking my doctors for help for years, but to no avail. We finally sat down and discussed everything. I then went to a new OB/GYN and once again asked for help. She recommended Astroglide, Prozac, DHEA and counseling.*
>
> *Over time we tried it all and today we have a very good sexual relationship. But we missed out on at least three years due to lack of knowledge about what we could do. I don't believe either of us would have opted to skip chemo just for me to be sexually responsive, but it*

Sexuality After Cancer Treatment

would have been very helpful to know what to expect before chemo started, then to get help dealing with the side effects without having to wait three years."

This patient's experience sums up the physical, psychological and relational struggles patients often face after cancer treatment ends.

Validation of Focus Group Findings

In 2010, the *Journal of Cancer Survivorship* reviewed 1,140 articles that had been written concerning the most common problems cancer patients experienced after cancer treatment. This literature review summarized and identified the major sexual issues impacting breast cancer survivors, which were the same issues we had discovered during our focus groups.

Major Sexual Side Effects Identified:

- Changes in body image associated with the loss of a breast
- Changes in body image associated with weight gain after cancer treatment
- Decreased sex drive related to chemotherapy drugs
- Increased vaginal dryness related to chemotherapy drugs
- Increased painful intercourse related to vaginal dryness from chemotherapy drugs
- Difficulty with arousal and orgasm related to cancer treatment
- Concern over future fertility related to chemotherapy

The *Journal of Cancer Survivorship* then identified the characteristics of patients who suffered the greatest impact on their sexual functioning.

Greatest Impact on Sexual Functioning Occurred In:

- Premenopausal women who received chemotherapy and did not have their menstrual periods return (remained menopausal)
- Women who experienced relational distress with their sexual partner
- Patients who were depressed and did not receive treatment for depression
- Patients who were treated with antidepressants for their depression (many antidepressants decrease sex drive)
- Patients who experienced decreased arousal and had difficulty achieving orgasm

CHAPTER 1

Hopefully, you are getting this book before you experience problems, and, if they should occur, you will know the interventions you can take to deal with them. Even if you have been dealing with sexual side effects for years, you can still address the problems. It is not too late. In later chapters, we will discuss each of the potential problems that the *Journal of Cancer Survivorship* identified and suggest interventions you can try. Restoring your sexual functioning after cancer treatment can become a reality.

Remember

- *Chemo-treated women experience a number of lingering side effects that directly impact their sexual functioning.*
- *The* Journal of Cancer Survivorship *found that 71 percent of surveyed cancer-treated women experienced sexual dysfunction after treatment was over. If you are experiencing sexual problems, you are not alone.*
- *Loss of sexual desire is a common cancer treatment side effect that impacts a majority of women.*
- *If you are blaming yourself for sexual problems you have encountered, STOP. The decrease in your previous sexual drive is not your fault!*
- *Sex is a normal part of life, but it is a topic most people feel uncomfortable discussing.*
- *The vast majority of doctors and nurses depend on the patient to initiate a discussion on the subject of sex. During routine appointments, let your healthcare provider know you have questions about sexuality.*
- *Approach the subject of sexuality with your physician. This allows your physician the opportunity to either answer your questions or refer you to another physician.*
- *Answers are available to help you regain your normal sexual functioning. Keep asking and seeking. The goal is to get your questions answered. Do not suffer without taking all steps necessary to find the help you need. You may need to talk to several healthcare providers before you receive the help you need.*
- *It is never too late to address the majority of problems that impact your quality of life and sexual functioning after cancer treatment. There are solutions to reduce or eliminate most of your problems.*

Chapter 2

Factors Affecting Sex Drive

As we begin this journey of understanding how to restore your sexual functioning, it is important to have a clear understanding of the factors that have a direct impact on your sex drive. We have discussed the fact that cancer treatment impacts sexual functioning, but it is not the only impacting factor that can directly contribute to decreased sex drive.

Sexual problems are often viewed as only a physical problem. The emphasis is placed on the performance "between the sheets." In reality, sexual functioning is a complex combination of a variety of impacting factors inside and outside of the body.

An individual's sex drive is determined by a combination of contributing factors—**physical**, **psychological**, **relational** and **cultural beliefs**. Sex drive is a complex interaction where our body meets up with our mind, our past experiences, our beliefs and our current relationship. Each of these contributing factors has an impact on how a woman feels about herself and determines her level of sexual desire. When even one of these contributing factors is weak or nonfunctional, sex drive diminishes.

To successfully address and restore your optimal sexual functioning, all influencing factors need to be assessed. There are factors, not related to chemotherapy, that can sabotage your sex life. In this chapter, we will discuss these factors.

Physical (Biological) Factors

A combination of physical factors directly impacts a woman's sex drive. It is essential to look carefully at all of the following physical causes that can decrease desire. Some causes are directly under your control and you

Chapter 2

can make changes or modifications to them. Other causes may require intervention by a healthcare provider to reduce or eliminate the impact.

Fatigue

Recovering from the physical fatigue of cancer surgery and chemotherapy is a frequent cause of low sexual desire. Gaining your energy back after surgery and chemotherapy is a gradual process. It does not happen quickly. It may take many months. Most patients report that it took them about a year after treatment ended to regain their normal level of vitality. When an individual is tired, sexual desire and sexual thoughts become a low priority. This is normal. Fatigue reduces desire in all areas of life.

If you are experiencing fatigue, you are among the vast majority of cancer treated women. Fatigue is the number one complaint of cancer patients during and after treatment. In the following chapters, we will discuss many of the contributing factors that can impact your energy and share what you can do to decrease their impact. In the meantime, know that you are normal if you are having a problem regaining your energy.

Hormones

Hormones regulate much of female sexual functioning. Reduced levels of all hormones in the body, especially after chemotherapy, have the greatest impact on reducing the sex drive. Chemotherapy causes the levels of all of the sex hormones to plummet. For premenopausal patients, this is apparent by the irregularity or cessation of the monthly period. The reduction of these hormones puts a woman in a temporary or permanent menopausal state. In this state, women experience the various symptoms of menopause. Younger women usually regain their hormonal functioning after treatment ends, but may continue to experience menstrual irregularities and may face an earlier menopause. Women nearer the age of natural menopause may remain in a menopausal state after treatment ends. Thus, chemotherapy-treated women have to deal with early menopausal symptoms and body changes.

Reduction in the hormone estrogen causes the majority of complaints for chemotherapy-treated patients. These complaints include hot flashes, night sweats, mood swings, vaginal dryness, depression, brain fog, sleeplessness, vaginal itching, painful intercourse and urinary changes. Reduction in the hormone testosterone greatly influences the sex drive.

Factors Affecting Sex Drive

Each of these individual changes will be discussed in detail in later chapters.

Medications

Medications, both over-the-counter and prescription, can promote fatigue and cause decreased sexual desire. Some antidepressants used to treat depression can cause a great reduction in both desire and in the ability to experience an orgasm. A list of medications that can reduce your sexual drive is provided in *Chapter 14: Drugs That Lower Your Sex Drive*.

Recreational drugs such as narcotics, stimulants and hallucinogens also affect sexual function. Low sexual desire, decreased arousal and lack of orgasm are results of recreational drug dependence.

Psychological Factors

Psychological or mental factors greatly impact a woman's sexual desire. You may have heard the saying, *"The mind is the most important sex organ."* This saying makes a very valid point, but ignores other circumstantial and physical factors that a woman treated with chemotherapy, or who has undergone menopause, may face. Throughout this book, we will explore the psychological factors of anxiety, depression, stress, body image, self-esteem and sexual history. These factors directly impact one's mental state, which can lower one's sexual desire.

Body Image

It is common for patients to struggle with physical self-esteem issues caused by cancer treatment. Surgery alters a woman's body image. An even greater body image impact occurs during chemotherapy. When a patient loses her hair and experiences the side effects of chemotherapy, it can cause severe body image issues.

Most body image issues, such as hair loss, weight gain or weight loss, are resolved by the passing of time after treatment ends. However, if a woman has had a mastectomy and has not undergone reconstruction, body image issues may continue.

Chapter 2

Body Image Change During Treatment

- 33% body image reduction **after surgery**
- 50% body image reduction **during** chemotherapy treatment
- 31% body image reduction **six months after** chemotherapy completion
- 24% body image reduction **one year after** treatment completion

— *EduCare Focus Group*

Low Body Image After Breast Surgery

Nudity becomes problematic for some women after breast surgery, especially if they have had a mastectomy. Some women resort to dressing and undressing in the dark to avoid having their partner see their surgically altered body. In our focus groups, six percent of women had never allowed their sexual partner to see their surgical scar. In order for the sexual relationship to return to as near normal as possible, dealing with the missing or altered breast is essential.

If you had a mastectomy and did not have reconstruction, a well-fitting prosthesis is essential. Make an appointment with a prosthesis consultant. Take a tight-fitting t-shirt with you to the appointment. Trying the t-shirt on over the prosthesis will allow you to see what it looks like under your clothes. It may also be helpful to take a friend along to provide honest feedback about the appearance of the prosthesis. Lacy, feminine bras with specially designed pockets to securely hold the prosthesis in place are available. Insurance covers the basic cost of the prosthesis and bras. Give the prosthesis consultant the name of your insurance provider and she will be able to tell you how much your policy covers for these purchases.

While at the prosthesis shop, ask about purchasing a light-weight temporary prosthesis that can be sewn into a lacy camisole or lingerie. You may also want to purchase a camisole with a pocket designed to hold soft fiberfill or your own prosthesis. Some women find that wearing a camisole with their prosthesis allows them to participate in sex without having to bare their chest. This increases their willingness to participate in sex without embarrassment. It is interesting to note that most sexual partners do not have their sexual interest diminished by the surgical change. It is most often the patient that is impacted.

Factors Affecting Sex Drive

Reconstruction After Breast Surgery

Often, patients are so overwhelmed with surgical and treatment decisions during diagnosis that they choose not to have reconstruction. Women who undergo breast reconstruction and have their body image restored, generally experience less anxiety and distress caused by nudity. If you did not choose to have breast reconstruction after your breast surgery, reconstruction is still an option. Reconstruction can be performed years after breast surgery. Previous treatments, such as chest wall radiation, may limit your reconstruction options, but there are procedures available.

You can ask your treatment team for a reconstructive surgeon recommendation, ask a friend who has had reconstruction or do an Internet search. Call to schedule a consultation to discuss appropriate reconstruction options. A consultation is usually free, and the surgeon's staff will estimate all out-of-pocket costs for you. Ask to see pictures of women who have had the type of reconstruction you are considering. You may wish to consult more than one surgeon about your options before making your final decision. For additional reconstruction information, refer to *Appendix A: Comparison of Breast Reconstruction Procedures* on page 173.

Weight Gain

Weight gain during cancer treatment is common for breast cancer patients. Some women feel that they are not as sexually attractive to their partner after weight gain and will avoid sexual activity for this reason. It is important to know that sexual partners are not usually as concerned about your weight as you are. It may be helpful if you share your concerns about your weight gain with your sexual partner. Most women find what a partner most desires is joyful, willing participation and excitement about the sexual activity.

Be cautious when choosing a diet for weight control. Weight control should always focus on providing the body with proper nutrition to build good health while cutting excess empty calories. Fad weight-loss diets are not recommended. While fad diets may work, they are usually stressful and frequently cut out food groups that are needed to ensure that your body is receiving proper nutrients to build and maintain your health. *Chapter 12: Value of Nutrition* will provide healthy eating tips to address weight issues.

Chapter 2

If you have gained weight due to cancer treatments, you can compensate by focusing on what you can control. The following tips can boost your self-esteem and help you feel more sexually attractive.

Tips To Boost Body Image:
- Get a new haircut
- Have a makeup consultation; update your makeup
- Update your wardrobe to compensate for weight gain; accent your positive features
- Buy sexy clothes for lounging around the house
- Buy sexy lingerie
- Join a local gym
- Hire a personal trainer to help you get in shape
- Join Weight Watchers® for group support (now available online)

Sexual History

Some women may experience problems with their current sexuality due to a history of traumatic sexual experiences such as rape or sexual abuse. These issues require the help of a trained professional to work through the deep psychological wounds. After a cancer diagnosis, it is not uncommon for women to experience a resurgence of emotional turmoil that they thought was forgotten and had been successfully managed. If you were a victim of sexual abuse and have never worked through the emotional impact with a professional, contact your healthcare facility or search the Internet for licensed professionals in your area who deal with sexual abuse. Seeking help is a wise decision for you and your family.

Relational Factors

Low sex drive can be greatly impacted by interpersonal problems in a relationship. For most women, emotional closeness or emotional intimacy is an essential prelude needed to create a desire to become sexually intimate with another individual. The emotional relationship with a sexual partner is of high importance to the majority of women. Therefore, stress or relationship problems can be a major contributing factor to low sexual desire. Relationship factors that greatly increase stress and reduce attraction to a partner will also be discussed in later chapters.

Factors Affecting Sex Drive

Cultural Belief Factors
We learn from our family of origin, and past life experiences the beliefs that shape our view of sexuality and how we should act today. "Norms" about relationships and intimacy were part of the beliefs we learned while growing up and we carry them into our present sexual relationships. Occasionally, these cultural norms promoted the belief that sex is only for procreation and is not to be found pleasurable by a female. If you have found that your beliefs about sexuality interfere with your enjoyment of sex, talking about these issues with a counselor may be helpful.

Exploring All Barriers to Sexual Functioning
In looking at sexual functioning after cancer treatment, it is essential to look at all aspects that can impact sexual desire. No stone can be left unturned if you are to discover what issues may be blocking or hindering your return to your previous level of sexual functioning. Since sexual desire is impacted by physical, psychological, relational and cultural beliefs, you have to look carefully at each area of your life to determine your individual influences. In my experience, it is usually a combination of issues that need to be addressed. My goal is to help you discover what is creating barriers and to help you learn what you can do to get your sexual enjoyment back.

Chapter 2

Personal Quality of Life Pre-Assessment
Where Do You Stand Today?

Complete the assessment on the following page. Rate your present state or condition in each area using the following scale:

1 = None/Little/Never/Low/No problem
(Does not interfere with quality of life)

3 = Occasional/Minimal/Tolerable
(Moderately interferes with quality of life)

5 = Severe/Very Frequent/High
(Severely interferes with quality of life)

When you review the completed assessment, factors that may impact your sexual functioning and overall quality of life will be identified. Each factor will be discussed in following chapters, along with interventions to help you reduce or eliminate the problem.

There will be a *Personal Quality of Life Post-Assessment* on page 166 to reevaluate your quality of life and sexual functioning after reading this book and implementing self-care recommendations. Completing the post-assessment will help you identify areas that need additional intervention.

Factors Affecting Sex Drive

Personal Quality of Life Assessment: Pre-Assessment	
Physical Symptoms	**Level of Distress**
Fatigue	(None) 1 2 3 4 5 (Severe)
Headaches	1 2 3 4 5
Hot Flashes	1 2 3 4 5
Night Sweats	1 2 3 4 5
Anxiety/Nervousness	1 2 3 4 5
Depression	1 2 3 4 5
Insomnia	1 2 3 4 5
Vaginal Dryness	1 2 3 4 5
Painful Intercourse	1 2 3 4 5
Loss of Sexual Libido	1 2 3 4 5
Weight Gain	1 2 3 4 5
Pain	1 2 3 4 5
Urine Leakage	1 2 3 4 5
Relationship Assessment	**Level**
Significant Other	☐ Good ☐ Stressful ☐ Very Stressful
Immediate Family	☐ Good ☐ Stressful ☐ Very Stressful
Close Friends	☐ Good ☐ Stressful ☐ Very Stressful
Social Life	☐ Good ☐ Stressful ☐ Very Stressful
Sexual Assessment	**Level**
Sex Drive (Libido)	☐ Good ☐ Low ☐ Very Low
Orgasm Ability	☐ Always ☐ Occasional ☐ Never
Body Image Assessment	**Level**
Physical Appearance	☐ Good ☐ Acceptable ☐ Unacceptable
Weight	☐ Good ☐ Acceptable ☐ Unacceptable
Overall Assessment	**Level**
Quality of Life: Physical	(Good) 1 2 3 4 5 (Poor)
Quality of Life: Psychological	1 2 3 4 5
Quality of Life: Relational	1 2 3 4 5

Chapter 2

Remember

- *You **deserve** to have your sexual functioning restored after cancer treatment. Your complete healing should include sexual healing.*
- *The first step is to investigate what may be contributing to or causing your reduction in sex drive.*
- *Causes for lack of desire are unique for each person. There may be a combination of causes, including physical, psychological, relational or cultural beliefs.*
- *There are interventions to address most causes of low sex drive.*
- *Together, we will explore how these influencing factors impact you and what you can do to get your sex life back.*

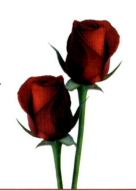

Chapter 3

Female Sexual Anatomy

As you work toward restoring your sexual functioning, it is very helpful to understand the basic sexual anatomy of the female body. Understanding the names and functions of the major anatomical parts that play a major part in female satisfaction will be helpful in our discussion of how to restore optimal sexual functioning.

External Female Anatomy

The external genitals are called the vulva. The vulva includes all of the external structures of the female anatomy, including the labia majora, labia minora, clitoris and vaginal opening (orifice).

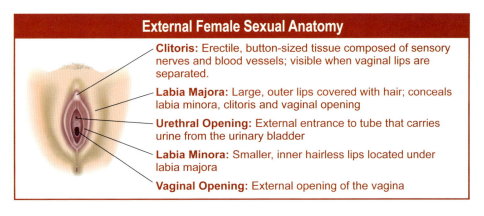

External Female Sexual Anatomy

Clitoris: Erectile, button-sized tissue composed of sensory nerves and blood vessels; visible when vaginal lips are separated.

Labia Majora: Large, outer lips covered with hair; conceals labia minora, clitoris and vaginal opening

Urethral Opening: External entrance to tube that carries urine from the urinary bladder

Labia Minora: Smaller, inner hairless lips located under labia majora

Vaginal Opening: External opening of the vagina

Clitoris

The Greek word for the clitoris is "key." The clitoris is the erectile portion of the female genitals and is the most sensitive female body part for creating arousal. Direct or indirect stimulation of the clitoris causes the sensory nerves to send a message to the brain that produces sexual arousal throughout the body. The clitoris is estimated to have 8,000 sensory nerve endings, more than any other part of the female body.

Chapter 3

Clitoral Complex Anatomy

Clitoral Glans: External, small button-sized erectile tissue composed of nerves and blood vessels; most sexually stimulating part of the female to create sexual arousal

Clitoral Crus: V-shaped, internal erectile tissue composed of nerves and blood vessels; extending from each side of external clitoral glans

Urethral Opening

Clitoral Bulbs: Internal erectile tissue that extends from both sides of the external gland and surrounds the urethral and vaginal orifices; during sexual stimulation they engorge with blood, creating a tight cuff around the vaginal orifice

Vaginal Opening

The clitoris is a wish-bone shaped dense network of spongy erectile tissue composed of blood vessels and nerves. The only visible part of the clitoris is a small, button-shaped portion called the glans of the clitoris. Most of the clitoris lies internally under the skin. The external and internal components of the clitoris are called the clitoral complex.

The visible portion (glans) of the female clitoris is located near the front junction of the labia minora (smaller, inner lips) and the opening of the urethra (urinary tube). It is composed of a dense network of erectile tissues and nerves. The visible glans of the clitoris is hidden under a type of hood (prepuce) formed when the thinner portions of the labia minora come together at the top of the glans. The hood protects the external glans from constant stimulation.

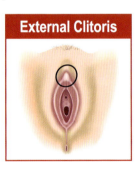
External Clitoris

The external glans of the clitoris branches internally into a wish-bone shape with two crus (leg-like extensions) that lie under the skin of the labia minora in a V-shape. These internal crus extend for about four inches on each side of the visible glans of the clitoris. In addition to the legs, there are two clitoral bulbs (vestibular) composed of erectile tissue that lie under the smaller lips. The entire clitoral complex has a complex network of sensory

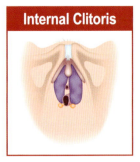
Internal Clitoris

Female Sexual Anatomy

nerves and blood vessels that fill with blood causing engorgement of the tissues when stimulated.

When the external or internal clitoral tissues are stimulated through direct or indirect touch, the clitoral nerves send signals to the spinal column that travel quickly to the brain. The brain then automatically sets off numerous changes throughout the body. The entire clitoral complex fills with blood. Blood flow to the labia, clitoris and vagina increases causing engorgement of the tissues.

Engorgement From Sexual Arousal Causes:

- External glans of the clitoris to becomes erect
- Clitoral hood to retract, exposing the visible glans
- Clitoral bulbs to form a firm, cuff-like enclosure surrounding the entrance to the vagina, which increases pleasure for the sexual partner
- Vaginal canal to lengthen
- Vaginal wall to increase secretion of a thin, slippery fluid which lubricates the vaginal canal and makes penetration more comfortable
- Breasts to increase in size and become more sensitive to touch
- Nipples to become erect and the areola to darken in color

Stimulation of the clitoris also creates other physiological changes in the body, including increased heart rate, increased blood pressure and flushing of the chest and upper body.

Female Clitoris Compared to Male Penis

The female clitoris and the male penis originate from the same hormonally-sensitive tissue. When an embryo is in the developmental stage in the uterus, the same hormone-sensitive tissue is present in both male and female babies. While in the uterus, a change occurs, and a baby boy's testicles begin producing the male hormone testosterone, and the hormone-sensitive tissue develops into a penis.

The major differences between males and females in these sexually-sensitive tissues (clitoris and penis) are the external size and urine flow. Externally, the male penis is much larger than the external portion of the clitoris. The majority of the clitoral tissues lie under the skin surrounding the vaginal opening. The female clitoris, unlike the male penis, does not connect to the urethra and is not involved in the urinary flow. The male

Chapter 3

penis has a urethral tube running through its entire length which expels urine during urination and sperm during ejaculation. The one common factor is that the male penis and the female clitoris are the most sexually-sensitive tissues in a person's body. Stimulation of either the clitoris or the penis results in sexual arousal.

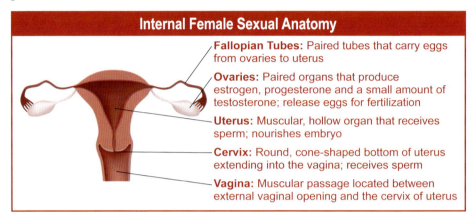

Internal Female Sexual Anatomy

Fallopian Tubes: Paired tubes that carry eggs from ovaries to uterus

Ovaries: Paired organs that produce estrogen, progesterone and a small amount of testosterone; release eggs for fertilization

Uterus: Muscular, hollow organ that receives sperm; nourishes embryo

Cervix: Round, cone-shaped bottom of uterus extending into the vagina; receives sperm

Vagina: Muscular passage located between external vaginal opening and the cervix of uterus

The Vagina

The vagina is a tube-like tunnel starting under the folds of the labia and ending at the cervix of the uterus. The vagina has two main functions: sexual intercourse and serving as the birth canal for childbirth. The walls of the vagina are composed of muscular tissues that have a high level of elasticity, which allows them to stretch and contract. During

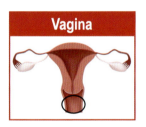

Vagina

either intercourse or childbirth, the vagina can stretch to the needed size and then return to its original size. During the resting state, the vagina collapses in on itself. The vaginal wall has a rough texture, which creates friction and stimulates the penis during intercourse, making vaginal intercourse pleasurable for the male partner. Engorgement and fluid secretion for vaginal lubrication allow intercourse to be pleasurable for both partners.

The vagina has few sensory nerves compared to the clitoris. In the vagina, the sensory nerves are concentrated in the lower one-third portion. The lower portion of the vagina, because of its concentration of sensory nerves, allows a pleasurable sensation during intercourse by rhythmically

Female Sexual Anatomy

contracting every eight-tenths of a second during orgasm. There are few sensory nerves in the remaining two-thirds of the vaginal wall.

The vagina is like any other body part with muscles; it will atrophy (gradually waste away) if it is not used on a regular basis. Non-use causes the muscles of the vaginal wall to lose their tone and reduce the blood supply needed for sexual arousal. Therefore, a healthy vagina needs regular use to remain fit and tone. The old saying "if you don't use it, you will lose it" applies to the female vagina. The regular increase of blood flow through sexual arousal or intercourse helps maintain the sexual health of the vagina.

What is the Vaginal "G-Spot"?

You may have heard of the "G-spot." It was named "G" after the doctor who first described it, Dr. Ernst Grafenberg. The "G-spot" refers to an area located under the pubic bone in the lower vaginal wall, located one to three inches from the vaginal opening on the side of the urinary bladder. Just as the clitoris is compared to the penis, the "G-spot" is often compared to the male prostate gland. The button-sized area is claimed to be extremely sensitive to deep stimulation resulting in sexual pleasure. Some also claim that the "G-spot" ejaculates fluid during orgasm.

For years, the "G-spot" has been one of the most debated areas of female sexual medicine by medical professionals. Some claim the existence of this area, while others refute the existence. Imaging studies are ongoing to further investigate the existence.

Vaginal Lubrication and Elasticity

Vaginal lubrication and elasticity of the vagina are directly under the influence of the female hormone estrogen. When estrogen levels are adequate, the vaginal wall cells are abundant, soft and elastic. The vaginal elasticity allows the vagina to stretch easily during intercourse without causing pain. Normal estrogen levels are also necessary for the vaginal wall to secrete lubricating fluid during sexual arousal. This lubricating fluid causes a female to feel wet. Lubrication increases sexual pleasure by making penetration more comfortable. When estrogen levels are low, the lubrication process is decreased and tissues that line the vagina become very thin, which causes vaginal dryness to increase. Vaginal dryness

Chapter 3

makes sexual intercourse uncomfortable and even painful. Extreme vaginal dryness causes pain during penetration and can result in bleeding after intercourse.

Estrogen levels significantly influence vaginal health. Since chemotherapy greatly reduces the amount of estrogen, vaginal dryness and lack of vaginal lubrication are problems common to most chemo-treated women. We will discuss how to deal with vaginal dryness and lack of lubrication in *Chapter 5: Vaginal Dryness and Painful Intercourse*.

Anatomy of the Uterus

The uterus is a muscular, pear-shaped organ that is approximately three to four inches long. It is located behind the urinary bladder, which is in front of the rectum and in the middle of the pelvis. The uterus is anchored in position by several ligaments. The main function of the uterus is to carry a developing fetus. The internal portion of the uterus prepares a thick vascular lining each month in preparation to nourish a fertilized egg. If an egg is not fertilized, this thickened vascular lining sheds monthly as the menstrual flow. The uterus does not play a major role in sexual arousal or pleasure.

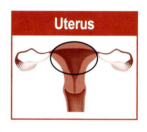

Anatomy of the Cervix

The cervix is the round, cone-shaped, lower part of the uterus. It extends into the vagina and has glands that produce mucus. This mucus, which is thick in consistency, helps sperm swim to a woman's egg during ovulation. It also acts as a barrier to prevent harmful microorganisms from entering the uterus and causing an infection.

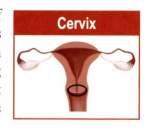

Increasing Sexual Satisfaction After Cancer Treatment

Chemotherapy reduces the hormones that drive your sexual pleasure and desire. Hormones are like a battery, which keeps the sexual organs charged. Chemotherapy causes a woman's hormonal battery to be low, providing a weak charge to the sexually-sensitive tissues. Because of this, most women experiencing treatment-induced menopause require more sexual stimulation to experience sexual pleasure or an orgasm. The key

Female Sexual Anatomy

to increasing your future sexual pleasure is to understand the functions of the clitoris and vagina.

The vagina is often mistaken to be the source of sexual pleasure. This misdirected focus is the reason many women do not reach orgasm during vaginal intercourse. It is estimated that 20 percent of women receiving vaginal stimulation only are able to experience an orgasm. Before chemotherapy, when your sex hormones were higher, stimulation to the vagina through penetrative intercourse only may have been adequate to promote orgasm. Now that your sex hormones are lower, vaginal intercourse alone may not provide the adequate nerve stimulation needed to promote pleasure and orgasm.

Although the vagina has abundant sexually-sensitive tissues, it does not have the same high degree as the clitoris. Remember, the clitoris contains about 8,000 sensory nerve endings, more than any other part of the female body. Without adequate clitoral stimulation, the potential to achieve the highest level of sexual satisfaction is reduced.

Most women require stimulation to the clitoris during intercourse to reach an orgasm. However, some women find direct stimulation to the clitoris to be uncomfortable and may prefer stimulation to the tissues surrounding the clitoris instead. Share this information with your partner to maximize your sexual pleasure.

Impact of the Mind on Sexuality

Now that we have discussed the functional role of different anatomical parts of the female anatomy, let's consider another major organ that impacts sexual function—the mind. As mentioned before, you have probably heard the saying, *"The mind is the most important sex organ."* This saying is a partial truth. The mind is necessary for full arousal and sexual pleasure; however, the full truth is that the mind is under the direct influence of sex hormones, psychological factors and physical factors that determine whether a person can experience full sexual pleasure. Physical and mental components are essential for pleasurable sex.

In this chapter, the focus has been on sexual anatomy and the physical functions of sex. However, for a female, both the physical and mental factors that influence sexual desire must be evaluated to restore pleasurable sexual function. These influencing factors vary widely among women. There is

Chapter 3

not a one-size-fits-all prescription to fix sexual dysfunction after cancer treatment. Instead, sexual restoration requires a personal evaluation and identification of your unique influencing factors so you can address them. In later chapters, we will discuss the influencing factors that can block your sexual pleasure and what you can do to eliminate or reduce their impact.

Female Sexual Anatomy

Remember

- *Understanding how different parts of female sexual anatomy function during sex helps you to maximize your sexual satisfaction.*
- *The clitoris is the most sensitive female sexual organ. It is the female organ equivalent to the male penis. The clitoris is the key to female sexual arousal. It has the largest number of sensory nerves in the body. Adequate stimulation of the clitoris during foreplay and intercourse are necessary to ensure sexual pleasure.*
- *The internal vaginal wall has far less sensory nerves than the external clitoris. The vaginal opening has sensory nerves in the lower one-third, but the remainder of the vagina has few sensory nerves. Thus, the vagina is not the most sensitive sexual area of the female anatomy to promote pleasure and orgasm.*
- *After cancer treatment, there are many influencing factors that can block your return to a satisfying sexual relationship. Physical and mental influencing factors must be assessed to determine potential causes that prevent you from restoring your sexual relationship.*

Chapter 4
Effect of Hormones on Sexuality

Hormones are the spark plugs of our life. We can't see them. They are invisible to the human eye; yet, every minute of the day, our quality of life is determined by their presence and their delicate balance.

Hormones are chemical substances produced by endocrine glands, such as the ovaries, adrenal glands or thyroid glands. The chemical substance they produce travels through body fluids to a distant organ where they find a receptor that allows them to enter the cells. After entering the cells of an organ, they cause an effect on the organ's functioning.

In this chapter, we are going to discuss the major sex hormones which may be influencing your sexuality and your quality of life after cancer treatment—estrogen, progesterone and testosterone. We will also briefly discuss thyroid hormone, a master hormone that influences many of the functions in your body.

Estrogen Hormone
There are three types of estrogen that can be found in a female at different stages of her life: estradiol, estrone and estriol.

- **Estradiol**: The primary estrogen during the menstrual years; causes the development of female characteristics at puberty and maintains the menstrual cycle
- **Estrone:** The primary estrogen produced after menopause; a much weaker type of estrogen; becomes the dominant estrogen after menopause
- **Estriol:** The estrogen produced mainly during pregnancy

In this book, we will refer to estradiol as estrogen for simplicity since it is the primary estrogen that causes sexual problems.

CHAPTER 4

The Role of Estrogen

The hormone estrogen (estradiol) made in the ovaries is responsible for the development of female characteristics. Most young girls begin to experience an upswing in estrogen production around 8 to 10 years of age. The first signs of this increase are perspiration and body odor. This is followed by the development of breast buds and the growth of pubic hair. Over the next several years, the breasts gradually increase in size, the vagina fully matures and the hips widen. During this time, most girls experience a weight gain of 20 – 30 pounds and a height increase of several inches in one year.

Full development of sex organs is evidenced by the onset of the menstrual period, which usually occurs 2.5 years after breast development with an average onset at 12 – 13 years of age.

Sources of Estrogen Production

Estrogen production occurs mainly in the ovaries. The ovaries produce about 90 percent of female estrogen. Another 10 percent is made in the body fat and skin from the conversion of other hormones (prohormones) androstenedione and dehydroepiandrosterone (DHEA). These hormones are circulating in the blood stream in an inactive form but can be converted into estrogen.

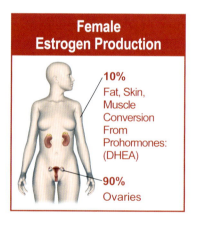

Female Estrogen Production

10% Fat, Skin, Muscle Conversion From Prohormones: (DHEA)

90% Ovaries

Progesterone

Progesterone is produced in the ovaries after the release of an egg mid cycle. Progesterone causes the lining of the uterus (endometrium) to secrete special proteins during the second half of the monthly cycle to increase the vascular (blood-filled) lining of the uterus. If a pregnancy occurs, progesterone is then produced by the placenta. Progesterone levels remain elevated throughout the pregnancy and are necessary to maintain the pregnancy.

Hormonal Cycling During the Menstrual Cycle

The two major hormones that control the menstrual cycle are estrogen and progesterone, which are mainly produced in the ovaries. After the onset

Effect of Hormones on Sexuality

of menstruation, a process of monthly hormonal cycling of estrogen and progesterone levels occur and continue through the reproductive years.

Each cycle length is between 28 – 30 days. During the first half of the cycle, estrogen levels increase to the highest level. Estrogen stimulates the buildup of the lining of the uterus, maintains the eggs in the ovaries and stimulates the release of an egg at midcycle. During the second half of the cycle, progesterone levels rise, which continues the uterine wall buildup to prepare it for implantation of a fertilized egg. If an egg is not fertilized, both estrogen and progesterone levels drop to their lowest levels and the lining of the uterus sheds causing the menstrual flow.

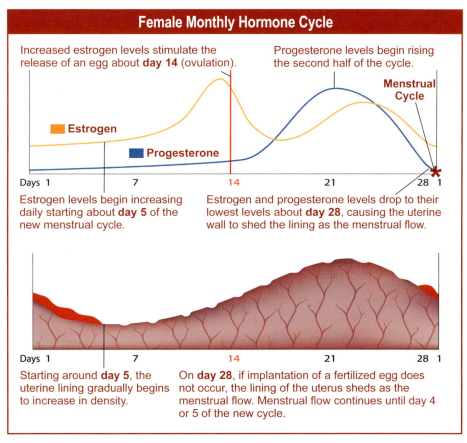

When estrogen and progesterone fall to their lowest levels the week before the menstrual period, women experience changes known as premenstrual syndrome (PMS). During this time, a woman may experience emotional

Chapter 4

changes that include anxiety, irritability, anger, poor concentration and crying spells. Physical changes may include headache, fatigue, weight gain from fluid retention, abdominal bloating, breast tenderness, muscle pain, joint pain and acne flare ups.

Most women have experienced some degree of PMS symptoms in the past when their hormones dropped to their lowest level a few days before menstruation. It is helpful to understand that PMS shares many symptoms experienced by chemo-treated women, but PMS symptoms are milder and last only for a few days.

Hormone Levels Control Menopausal Status

Estrogen and progesterone levels are predictors of your menopausal status. Hormone functioning determines if you are premenopausal, perimenopausal or postmenopausal.

- **Premenopausal:** Estrogen and progesterone levels cycle during the month within a range that produces a monthly menstrual period.
- **Perimenopausal:** Hormone levels begin to decline and fluctuate during the monthly cycle. Progesterone levels decrease first causing fertility to decline. Estrogen levels may fluctuate from low to high from cycle to cycle. High levels may range 20 – 30 percent higher than normal causing symptoms of painful or fibrocystic breasts, bloating, trouble sleeping, mood swings and changes in weight gain. Fluctuating levels may also cause the menstrual period to become irregular. The average time of the perimenopausal transition into menopause takes about 3.8 years.
- **Menopausal:** A period of 12 consecutive months with no menstrual period.

Post-Treatment Menopausal State

One of the common side effects experienced by premenopausal patients after chemotherapy treatments is the stopping of the menstrual cycle. This is proof that treatment has interrupted normal hormonal production. The common questions asked are, *"Will my menstrual period return?"* and *"If it does not return, what does this mean?"*

Many factors influence whether or not the menstrual period will return. These factors include the age of a patient, the medications used during treatment and a patient's unique personal physical functioning. Doctors cannot accurately predict who will have their periods return, or when it

Effect of Hormones on Sexuality

might happen. Because of the unique physical functioning of each woman, the same treatment can have a different response in different patients, complicating an accurate prediction by a physician. For younger women, hormonal function may return within several months after treatment ends. For other women, it may be a year or longer. Some women may experience permanent menopause. Different drug protocols may have greater impact on hormonal functioning than others.

Menstrual Period Return Factors:
- The younger a woman is when treated, the more likely her period will return.
- The closer a woman is to menopause, the more likely her period will not return.
- If the menstrual period does not return within 12 months, a woman will experience permanent menopause. A permanent menopausal state signals that the hormonal side effects and sexuality issues will continue.

Testosterone in Females

Many women are surprised to discover that functioning ovaries not only produce female hormones, but also produce testosterone, the predominant male hormone. However, the testosterone level in males is 10 – 20 times higher than in females. Females need testosterone for a healthy sex life. In a female, testosterone is the hormone that causes sexual desire and the biological sexual response necessary for arousal and orgasm. Testosterone is the hormone that propels a woman's sex drive by stimulating sexual thoughts, sparking sexual interest, causing the nipples and clitoris to be sensitive, and promoting orgasm.

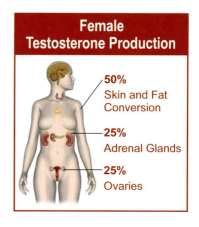

Female Testosterone Production

50% Skin and Fat Conversion

25% Adrenal Glands

25% Ovaries

The ovaries produce about 25 percent of a female's testosterone. The adrenal glands, located on top of the kidneys, produce approximately 25 percent. The remaining 50 percent is produced by the conversion of prohormones in the skin and fat. Testosterone is responsible for sex drive while estrogen is responsible for making intercourse comfortable.

Chapter 4

Estrogen keeps the lining of the vaginal walls soft, spongy and elastic, with the ability to provide lubrication during sexual stimulation. But, testosterone is the hormone that fuels female sexual desire, arousal and orgasm.

Role of Hormones

Estrogen:
- Promotes development of female characteristics
- Stimulates growth of breast tissue
- Maintains vaginal blood flow
- Promotes lubrication of vagina
- Thickens and keeps vaginal lining elastic
- Preserves bone density
- Promotes healthy urinary tract lining
- Induces ovulation and release of egg

Progesterone:
- Prepares lining of the uterus for a fertilized egg
- Helps maintain pregnancy

Testosterone:
- Plays a key role in women's estrogen production
- Promotes adult body odor, increased oiliness of skin, pubic and axillary hair growth
- Contributes to sexual drive, arousal and ability to experience an orgasm
- Helps maintain bone and muscle mass
- Levels highest in 20's; levels slowly decline with age; menopausal level is half of level during 20's

Thyroid Hormone Function

The thyroid gland is a butterfly-shaped gland in the neck that secretes two types of thyroid hormones that affect the function of virtually every organ in the body. Thyroid hormones control the speed of the chemical functions in the body (metabolism). They impact heart rate, skin maintenance, temperature regulation and digestion. Two of the most common thyroid disorders are hypothyroidism (too low) and hyperthyroidism (too high).

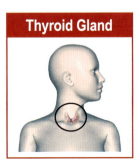
Thyroid Gland

Effect of Hormones on Sexuality

Hypothyroidism

Hypothyroidism is a frequent disorder in menopausal women who have undergone cancer treatment. The most common symptoms are fatigue and weight gain, which are caused by a slowed metabolism. Fatigue greatly impacts your quality of life and serves as a barrier to restoring your sexuality. If fatigue, combined with weight gain, is a problem, consider having your thyroid levels evaluated. Being tested for hypothyroidism is simple. Blood is drawn and sent to a laboratory for evaluation.

Symptoms of Hypothyroidism:

- Fatigue
- Concentration problems
- Feeling cold
- Muscle and joint aches
- Constipation
- Weight gain, despite diminished appetite
- Dry skin
- Coarse hair
- Hair loss
- Depression
- Eyebrows thinning (especially the last 1/3 of the brow)

If you are experiencing a combination of the listed symptoms, ask your physician to evaluate your thyroid function. Thyroid medication is available to bring thyroid levels back into normal levels and reverse the adverse symptoms.

Natural Versus Medically-Induced Menopause

Natural Menopause

Natural menopause is the process of a woman gradually losing her estrogen and progesterone production without surgical or chemical intervention. Over a period of years, the estrogen and progesterone made in her ovaries, as well as her androgens (testosterone and other male hormones) produced by the ovaries and adrenal glands gradually decline. Natural menopause allows a woman to **gradually** adjust to the reduction of sex hormones over a period of years (average of 3.8 years).

Estrogen loss causes the symptoms experienced during PMS to remain constant. Progesterone loss is mainly evidenced by the lack of fertility. The decline in androgens lowers the sex drive. Testosterone production continues in the ovaries for approximately six years after the loss of estrogen and progesterone. Research shows when menopause is reached,

Chapter 4

approximately 40 percent of menopausal women experience a decline in their sex drive.

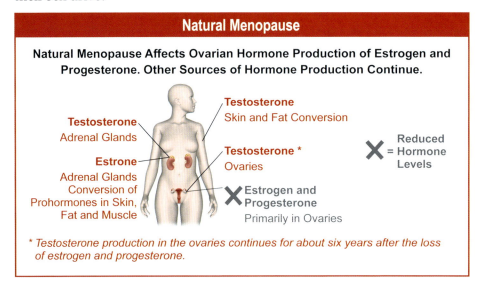

Medically-Induced Menopause

There is a significant difference between natural menopause and medically-induced menopause, caused by either surgical removal of the ovaries or by chemotherapy medications (often called chemopause). We discussed the process of natural menopause to prepare you to understand the difference in medically-induced menopause. Medically-induced menopause occurs very quickly, beginning the first day after the removal of the ovaries or with the first chemotherapy infusion.

Surgical menopause causes a premenopausal woman to enter the same hormonal state as a menopausal woman who loses hormonal production from her ovaries only. She maintains the hormonal functioning from other sources (adrenals, skin/fat conversion). However, she loses testosterone production from the ovaries.

Chemotherapy-induced menopause is vastly different because the drugs are systemic; they impact and reduce **all** sources of hormone production in the body (ovaries, adrenals and skin/fat conversion). Since all sources of hormone production are reduced after chemotherapy, it causes a greater intensity of symptoms.

Effect of Hormones on Sexuality

Women who are in natural menopause when beginning chemotherapy treatments experience fewer symptoms than premenopausal women when given the same drugs and dosages during treatment. However, their menopausal symptoms are intensified after chemotherapy.

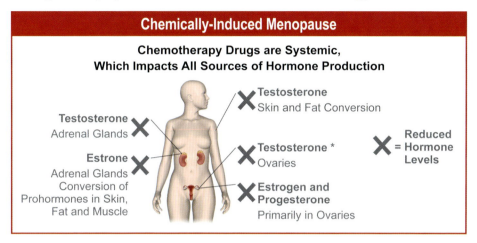

The Impact of Estrogen Loss

A common misconception is that loss of estrogen affects **only** the loss of fertility. Loss of estrogen not only ends fertility, but it also causes a number of problems throughout the body that impact a woman's quality of life.

Why does loss of estrogen cause so many problems? It is because estrogen receptors have been identified on over 300 tissues in the body. Estrogen plays a functioning role in many organs and tissues in the body. Dr. Benita S. Katzenellenbogen, a professor of physiology, cell and structural biology, has studied the hormone estrogen for decades. When ask if there was any part of the body that estrogen did not affect, she said *"I used to think so. Now I have my doubts. Well, maybe the spleen."*

It is now known that many organs and their functions are affected by estrogen. When estrogen levels decline, it not only affects fertility, but it also affects many organs in the body causing multiple symptoms throughout the body to occur. Intensity of symptoms vary among women. Some women experience multiple symptoms, which decreases their quality of life, while others may find their symptoms tolerable. Response to estrogen deprivation varies among women. The following graphic

Chapter 4

shows the major organs under estrogen influence and the symptoms that may manifest after estrogen reduction.

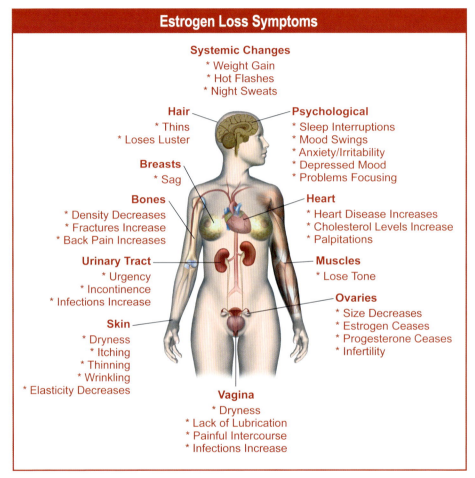

Impact of Estrogen Reduction on Sexuality

When a woman undergoes chemotherapy for cancer, the impact on her sex hormones is great. Estrogen hormone loss causes the majority of side effects experienced. The reduction in estrogen levels impacts many functions in the body and is experienced to some degree by all women undergoing cancer treatment.

The highest concentration of estrogen is found in the vulva tissues, the vaginal wall and in the muscles of the pelvis, bladder and urethra. Therefore, these tissues suffer the greatest impact after chemotherapy.

Effect of Hormones on Sexuality

After chemotherapy, most women experience some degree of vaginal dryness, pain and urinary changes. After cancer treatment is completed, medications prescribed for breast cancer estrogen receptor-positive cancers to prevent recurrence (aromatase inhibitor, tamoxifen) are designed to continue to reduce or block estrogen on these target tissues. These medications continue to cause side effects. Estrogen reduction can cause hot flashes, night sweats, palpitations of the heart, insomnia, fatigue, bone loss, mood swings and a loss of sexual drive. All the side effects caused by low estrogen levels impact your quality of life and can directly or indirectly interfere with your sex life.

Impact of Testosterone Reduction on Sexuality

During natural menopause, testosterone production in the ovaries continues for about six years after the loss of estrogen and progesterone. However, in chemically-induced menopause, the testosterone levels are impacted equally at the same time. Loss of testosterone causes a decrease in: sexual desire, genital and nipple sensitivity during foreplay, the ability to become sexually aroused and the ability to experience an orgasm.

Moving Forward

The most important fact to remember is that sexuality is hormonally driven, whether it be sexual desire, ability to have an orgasm or the ability to produce adequate vaginal lubrication to make intercourse comfortable. Without adequate levels of these sex hormones, our bodies revert to the pre-pubertal stage of a young girl with very little sexual interest or desire.

We end this chapter after introducing you to a quandary of side effects from chemotherapy. It is important to remember that chemotherapy has given long-term survival to millions of patients. Chemotherapy helped eradicate cancer, a potentially life-threatening disease, from your body. Hopefully, this chapter, though technical at times, has allowed you to understand how chemotherapy has caused side effects and how medically-induced menopause differs from natural menopause. Although the side effects after treatment may be bothersome, they are not life-threatening. In the following chapters, we will be discussing side effects in detail and providing you answers, along with self-care interventions to improve your quality of life.

Chapter 4

Remember

- *Hormones rule. Female hormones play a major role in how a woman feels and functions.*

- *Chemotherapy impacts the hormonal balance of a woman's body by greatly reducing sex hormones. The reduction in female hormones causes menopausal side effects. The most common menopausal side effects are hot flashes, night sweats, changes in mood, vaginal dryness, painful intercourse, urinary changes and sleep interruption.*

- *Hormonal reduction of testosterone can also lower sexual desire and decrease the ability to have an orgasm.*

- *Hormonal changes after cancer treatment may be temporary, or they may be long-lasting. It is difficult for a physician to predict the impact on an individual's hormonal functioning. The impact varies according to a woman's age, her menopausal status at the time of treatment, and the type and length of drugs administered. Some premenopausal women will regain their hormonal functioning after a period of time, while others may remain in a permanent menopausal state.*

- *Most side effects of chemotherapy have interventions that are effective in reducing or eliminating the impact on your quality of life.*

- *Another hormone, which is not a sex hormone, but impacts sexuality and is often neglected after cancer treatment, is thyroid hormone. Low thyroid function, hypothyroidism, is a common disorder in women that causes many symptoms impacting quality of life. If you are experiencing fatigue, constipation, weight gain, insomnia and are frequently feeling cold, ask to have your thyroid levels checked. An endocrinologist specializes in diagnosing and correcting hypothyroidism.*

- *Seek help in finding relief from the side effects you may be experiencing. You may have to visit several healthcare providers to find one who is skilled in managing menopausal side effects. Don't stop your search for answers. Keep looking. You deserve answers and help.*

Chapter 5

Vaginal Dryness and Painful Intercourse

One of the major problems menopausal and chemo-treated women experience is vaginal dryness. Adequate levels of estrogen keep the vaginal and external tissues soft, elastic and lubricated. When estrogen levels are too low to adequately nourish the cells, vaginal dryness occurs, which causes vaginal itching, increased potential for vaginal infections and painful intercourse. If the dryness is severe, bleeding after penetrative intercourse may also occur.

Vaginal Dryness

- 119% increase in vaginal dryness **during** treatment
- 131% increase in vaginal dryness **six months after** treatment completion
- 158% increase in vaginal dryness **one year after** treatment completion

Vaginal dryness is a continuing side effect experienced by most chemo-treated women.

— EduCare Focus Group Data

Vaginal dryness can be the side effect that has the greatest impact on restoring your sexual relationship. Correcting vaginal dryness is essential. There are a number of non-hormonal and hormonal treatments available to relieve the symptoms of vaginal dryness. Discovering the right product or combination of products to diminish your symptoms may take time.

Chapter 5

Patient Quotes

"I had so much vaginal dryness, I was afraid if I walked fast, I would crack my vagina."

"I started thinking my husband should find another partner because the one he had had completely dried up."

"We had intercourse without a lubricant and I was sore for a week."

"When I told my doctor, several months after finishing chemo, that I had bled after intercourse both times we tried, he responded 'Sounds like you're going to need Prozac to get through this.' I looked at him and said, 'Pardon me sir, but the problem is in my behind and not my head.' I left the office furious. We have not had intercourse for two years because my husband is afraid of hurting me again. I feel so sorry for him. We have only been married for three years. I have not mentioned my problem again to anyone until now."

— *Patient Quotes, EduCare Focus Group*

Painful Intercourse

- 137% increase in painful intercourse **during** treatment
- 147% increase in painful intercourse **six months after** treatment completion
- 163% increase in painful intercourse **one year after** treatment completion

Vaginal dryness and pain during penetrative intercourse continues to increase the first year after chemotherapy is completed. Pain is related to untreated vaginal dryness.

— *EduCare Focus Group Data*

In this chapter, we will describe the non-hormonal lubricants and moisturizers available to treat vaginal dryness symptoms. We will also describe the prescription hormonal products that can provide local relief, but are not systemic (affecting the entire body). These descriptions will help you in your search for the product or products that will meet your specific need. The goal is to start with the interventions that are non-hormonal to determine if you can achieve the relief you need. These products are available over-the-counter and do not require a healthcare provider's prescription. If you do not achieve the desired relief, you can then talk to your healthcare provider about the availability of prescription hormonal products that can provide additional relief.

Vaginal Dryness and Painful Intercourse

Treating Vaginal Dryness
Sexual functioning can only be successfully restored when you reduce the pain and discomfort caused by vaginal dryness and atrophy (thinning of the vaginal wall). The North American Menopause Society (NAMS) recommends that non-hormonal interventions, along with regular vaginal intercourse, be the first steps taken to reduce vaginal discomfort from estrogen loss.

Vaginal Lubricants
A vaginal lubricant is a gel or liquid applied to the vaginal canal and external genitals as a temporary measure to moisten the tissues during sexual intercourse. Lubricants are designed to reduce friction on the external vaginal lips and the internal vaginal tissues. Lubricants are successful in reducing local discomfort and pain caused by friction from foreplay, intercourse or the use of sex toys. A vaginal lubricant is not absorbed into the skin and is a temporary solution that increases sexual pleasure, but it has no long-term impact on restoring or maintaining moisture in the vaginal tissues.

Vaginal lubricants are available over-the-counter in the personal care section of the pharmacy. A wide selection is available, in a variety of formulas, making a first-time selection difficult. Selection of the correct lubricant is made based on your need. Lubricant formulas are either water-based, silicone-based or oil-based with each having advantages and disadvantages.

Lubricant Selection Precautions
- **Irritating Formulas:** Lubricants that contain glycerin or paraben may cause irritation or burning for some women. If you experience irritation after using a lubricant, select a different one that does not contain glycerin or paraben. If you continue to experience burning or itching, contact a healthcare provider to determine if you may have another condition contributing to the problem.
- **Condom Compatibility:** Some lubricants are not recommended when using a condom because they can increase slippage and breakdown the integrity of the condom. Oil-based vaginal lubricants have the potential to weaken the integrity of latex condoms. Tests conducted on condoms with an oil-based lubricant applied to them before pressurized

Chapter 5

air inflation had a higher burst rate than those without oil. Oil-based lubricants have also been shown to increase the slippage rate during intercourse. Water-based lubricants can also increase slippage rate, but do not contribute to the breakdown of the integrity of the condom. Therefore, oils or oil-based formulas are not recommended for use with latex condoms. Non-latex condoms are available. Most silicone or water-based formulas are compatible with condoms.

- **Sperm Viability:** Many lubricants can negatively affect sperm and slow motility (movement) even though they do not contain a spermicide. If you are trying to get pregnant, you should select a lubricant that does not damage or decrease the motility of sperm. Non-commercial products such as glycerin, olive oil, vegetable oil and even saliva have been associated with decreased sperm function in studies. The 2008 *"Effect of Vaginal Lubricants on Sperm Motility and Chromatin Integrity"* study found that Astroglide® and Replens® cause a dramatic decrease in sperm function because they change the pH of the vagina. The study found that the lubricant Pre-Seed® was found to maintain a normal pH level and is recommended for women desiring to get pregnant.

- **Specialty Lubricants:**
  - **Warming Lubricants** cause a heating sensation on the genitals. In contrast to products designed to reduce pain from vaginal dryness, these lubricants are marketed specifically for sexual enhancement. The heating sensation usually comes from the addition of menthol, L-arginine or capsaicin. These ingredients dilate blood vessels and cause a heating or cooling sensation. They have not been scientifically proven to enhance sexual function or promote orgasm. In fact, for a woman experiencing vaginal dryness, the added ingredients in the products can increase irritation and burning.
  - **Flavored Lubricants** are also available that contain added artificial flavors to improve taste. Because the added ingredients may have the potential to irritate sensitive vaginal tissues, it is recommended that you avoid flavored lubricants if you have dry vaginal tissues.

Natural Lubricants

For women who desire an all-natural lubricant, coconut oil has received rave reviews from women. At temperatures above 75 degrees, coconut oil is a liquid; below 75 degrees, it becomes a solid. If it is solid, it will quickly

Vaginal Dryness and Painful Intercourse

melt when applying to vaginal tissues. Coconut oil has properties of being antifungal, antiviral and antibacterial, which makes it an excellent lubricant for menopausal women to protect against vaginal infections. It is also an excellent daily moisturizer to be applied to the external genitals to reduce dryness. Coconut oil has a pleasant smell, tastes good and contains no harmful chemicals. Coconut oil can be purchased at health food stores and grocery stores at a lower price than commercial lubricants.

Olive oil is another natural lubricant that is inexpensive and readily available. Neither coconut oil nor olive oil is recommended as lubricants with latex condom use. These oils both have the potential to increase condom breakage.

Vaginal Lubricants Comparison Charts

A lubricant ingredient list is included in the following charts to allow you to determine which lubricant may be most suited for your need. You can determine if a lubricant will be irritating by trying a small patch test of the lubricant on your skin. If the skin shows no reaction after 24 hours, it should be safe to use.

	Silicone-Based Lubricants
ID Millennium®	**Ingredients:** Cyclomethicone, dimethicone
	Note: Less drying.
Pjur®	**Ingredients:** Cyclopentasiloxane, dimethicone, dimethiconol
	Note: Compatible with condoms.
Pink®	**Ingredients:** Dimethicone, vitamin E, aloe vera, dimethiconol, cyclomethicone
	Note: Compatible with condoms.
Astroglide X®	**Ingredients:** Cyclomethicone, dimethicone
	Notes: Waterproof and long lasting.

Chapter 5

	Water-Based Lubricants
Slippery Stuff®	**Ingredients:** Water, polyoxyethylene, methylparaben, propylene glycol, isopropanol
Astroglide®	**Ingredients:** Water, glycerin, methylparaben, propylparaben, polypropylene, glycol, polyquaternium, hydroxyethylcellulose, sodium benzoate **Notes:** Available in glycerin-free and paraben-free formulation
K-Y Jelly®	**Ingredients:** Water, glycerin, hydroxyethylcellulose, parabens, chlorhexidine
Summer's Eve®	**Ingredients:** Water, propylene glycol, methylcellulose, xanthan gum, sodium lactate, methylparaben, lactic acid, dextrose, sodium chloride, edatate disodium, pectin, propylparaben
FemGlide®	**Ingredients:** Water, polyoxyethylene, methylparaben, sodium carbomer
Just Like Me®	**Ingredients:** Water (Eau), glycerin, zanthan gum, hydroxyethylcellulose, methylparaben, potassium sorbate, disodium EDTA, sodium saccharin
Liquid Silk®	**Ingredients:** Purified Water, propylene glycol, isopropyl palmitate, dimethicone, cellulose polymer, polysorbate 60, sorbitan stearate, cetearyl alcohol, glyceryl Stearate NSE, B.N.P.D. Disodium EDTA, phenoxyethanol, methyl paraben, butyl paraben, ethyl paraben, propylparaben, BHT **Notes:** Formulated to be bio-static. When exposed to any bacteria, yeast infection or fungal spores, it will stop them from spreading.
Pre-Seed®	**Ingredients:** Water, hydroxyethylcellulose, arabinogalactan, paraben, Pluronic copolymers **Note:** Recommended for women who are trying to conceive.

Vaginal Dryness and Painful Intercourse

	Natural / Oil-Based Lubricants
Elegance Women's Lubricant®	**Ingredients:** Natural oils
	Notes: Does not contain alcohol, glycerin, or parabens; is compatible with a condom; helpful for women who have chronic vulva pain.
Olive Oil	**Ingredients:** Natural oil
	Notes: Inexpensive. Not recommended with condoms.
Coconut Oil	**Ingredients:** Natural oil
	Notes: Antibacterial and antifungal. Smells good. Inexpensive. Not recommended with condoms.

Vaginal Moisturizers

Vaginal moisturizers are often confused with vaginal lubricants. Vaginal moisturizers are like facial moisturizers; they help retain moisture in the tissues. They are **not** designed to be used as a lubricant for intercourse. A vaginal moisturizer reduces vaginal dryness as long as the moisturizer is regularly applied, usually several times a week. Vaginal moisturizers are formulated into a gel or cream to be applied to the vaginal tissues to maintain moisture. Although vaginal moisturizers are less effective than hormonally-based products, they have been shown to treat symptoms of vaginal dryness and significantly reduce discomfort during intercourse. Vaginal moisturizers are sold over-the-counter and do not require a prescription. You may wish to discuss the list on the following page with your healthcare provider to get a recommendation.

Chapter 5

	Vaginal Moisturizers
Replens®	**Ingredients:** Water, carbomer, polycarbophil, paraffin, hydrogenated palm oil, glyceride, sorbic acid, sodium hydroxide **Note:** Should be used 3 times weekly.
Moist Again®	**Ingredients:** Water, carbomer, aloe, citric acid, chlorhexidine deglutinate, sodium benzoate, potassium sorbate, diazolidnyl urea, sorbic acid **Note:** Safe to use with a latex condom; no data on effects on sperm motility.
Vagisil Feminine Moisturizer®	**Ingredients:** Water, glycerin, propylene glycol, poloxamer 407, methylparaben, polyquaternium-32, propylparaben, chamomile, aloe
Feminease®	**Ingredients:** Water, mineral oil, glycerin, yerba santa, cetyl alcohol, methyl paraben **Note:** Yerba santa, a plant native to the Pacific Northwest used as a moisturizer in place of aloe.
K-Y Long Lasting Moisturizer®	**Ingredients:** Purified water, glycerin, mineral oil, calcium/sodium PVM/MA copolymer, PVM/MA decadiene crosspolymer, hydrogenated palm glyceride, methylparaben, benzoic acid, tocopherol acetate, sodium hydroxide
K-Y Silk-E®	**Ingredients:** Water, propylene glycol, sorbitol, polysorbate 60, hydroxyethylcellulose, benzoic acid, methylparaben, tocopherol, aloe
Luvena Prebiotic Vaginal Moisturizer®	**Ingredients:** PEG, propanediol, purified water, jojoba oil, polypropylene glycol, cranberry extract, acesulfame-K, lysozyme, lactoferrin, lactoperoxidase, lactic acid, potassium thiocyanate, glycogen, d-mannose, vitamin E **Note:** Formulated with enzymes and proteins that may help keep bacteria and yeast in check.

Topical Vaginal Hormonal Therapies

Vaginal dryness occurs from a lack of the hormone estrogen. It is experienced after natural menopause, treatment with chemotherapy or when taking anti-hormonal drugs after breast cancer to reduce the risk of cancer recurrence. Women diagnosed with breast cancer who were determined to be estrogen receptor-positive are most often cautioned to

Vaginal Dryness and Painful Intercourse

avoid systemic estrogen therapy as a treatment for menopausal symptoms. It is recommended that estrogen receptor-positive women try vaginal lubricants and moisturizers as the first line of treatment for vaginal dryness.

For many women, the regular use of vaginal lubricants and moisturizers provides the relief needed to make intercourse and sexual activity more comfortable. However, for some women, not enough relief is provided with these interventions. Often, their vaginal dryness symptoms are accompanied by urinary symptoms of increased frequency, burning, urgency or leakage, which are also caused by low estrogen levels. Urinary symptoms occur because the cells that line the vaginal and urinary tract are no longer nourished and are not kept supple and moist by estrogen hormones. For women who do not find relief when using moisturizers and lubricants, the next step in finding symptom relief is with local, non-systemic (not affecting the entire body) local estrogen therapy.

Understanding Local Estrogen Therapy

Local, non-systemic estrogen therapy provides relief to the vagina, urinary tract and bladder tissues when applied inside the vagina. In about six weeks, 80 – 90 percent of patients report significant symptom improvement.

In studies of local estrogen therapy, the systemic blood level of estrogen increased when therapy was initiated but remained within menopausal range. In approximately four weeks, blood levels dropped back to the pre-treatment range, indicating therapy was not affecting the whole body.

The hormonal therapies described in this chapter contain low levels of estrogen that are administered locally to the vaginal area. These medications are absorbed locally and cause the vaginal and urinary tissues to replenish and mature. These new cells regain the ability to produce moisture. Within weeks, vaginal dryness and urinary symptoms begin to decrease. For most women, the symptoms are gone or are significantly decreased within twelve weeks. During this time, the estrogen in the blood level remains within the baseline (original) menopausal level.

Chapter 5

Types of Local Estrogen Therapy

Estrogen Vaginal Cream

Estrace®, Premarin® or Estragyn® is inserted into the vagina using a plastic applicator designed to measure the prescribed dosage accurately. Medication is usually inserted into the vagina twice a week, but scheduling may vary according to the severity of symptoms.

Estrogen Vaginal Cream
Local Hormonal Treatment for Vaginal and Urinary Symptoms

- **Premarin®**
  - **Pharmaceutical Formulation:** 0.5 g (0.625 mg/g of conjugated estrogen)
  - **Source of Active Ingredient:** Urine of pregnant mares
  - **Administration:** Insert 0.5 g daily for 3 weeks; then, twice weekly or as ordered by your healthcare provider
- **Estrace®**
  - **Pharmaceutical Formulation:** 0.1 mg of estradiol/g of cream
  - **Source of Active Ingredient:** Synthesized from soy and yams
  - **Administration:** Insert 0.5 g daily for 1 or 2 weeks; then, twice weekly or as ordered by your healthcare provider
- **Estragyn®**
  - **Pharmaceutical Formulation:** 2 – 4 g/d (1 mg active ingredient/g)
  - **Source of Active Ingredient:** Estrone
  - **Administration:** Insert daily for 1 – 2 weeks; then, twice weekly or as ordered by your healthcare provider

---

Estrogen Vaginal Tablet

Vagifem® is a plant-based estradiol tablet made from soy. It is inserted into the vagina daily for two weeks; then, the frequency is reduced to twice a week to maintain levels. In clinical studies comparing the Vagifem® tablet and vaginal cream, Vagifem® showed an 85.5 percent reduction of symptoms after twelve weeks, while the vaginal cream had a 41.4 percent reduction. Estrogen levels remain within postmenopausal levels.

Vaginal Dryness and Painful Intercourse

Estrogen Vaginal Tablet
Local Hormonal Treatment for Vaginal and Urinary Symptoms

- **Vagifem®**
  - **Pharmaceutical Formulation:** 25 mcg of estradiol
  - **Source of Active Ingredient:** Synthesized from soy
  - **Administration:** One tablet intravaginally daily for 2 weeks; then, twice weekly or as ordered by your healthcare provider

Estrogen Vaginal Ring

Estring® is a two-inch ring of estrogen derived from Mexican yams. It is inserted into the vagina and left in place. The estrogen ring has a silicone polymer cover that regulates a slow release of estrogen over a three-month period. Clinical studies show that Estring® has minimal systemic absorption. Estrogen levels remain within postmenopausal levels. Femring® is also an intravaginal ring of estrogen.

Estrogen Vaginal Ring
Local Hormonal Treatment for Vaginal and Urinary Symptoms

- **Estring®**
  - **Pharmaceutical Formulation:** 2 mg (delivers 6-9 mcg of estradiol daily)
  - **Source of Active Ingredient:** Synthesized from Mexican yams
  - **Administration:** Insert 1 ring intravaginally for 3 months or as ordered by your healthcare provider
- **Femring®**
  - **Pharmaceutical Formulation:** 0.05 milligrams (mg) a day and 0.1 mg a day
  - **Source of Active Ingredient:** Estradiol acetate
  - **Administration:** Intravaginal ring should remain in the vagina for 3 months or as ordered by your healthcare provider

Breast Cancer Patients' Concern

Many breast cancer patients hesitate to consider hormonal treatment for fear that they may cause their estrogen receptor-positive cancer to return. However, studies have shown that systemic estrogen levels stay within the menopausal range when local hormonal therapies are used to treat vaginal atrophy, dryness and urinary symptoms. If your cancer was estrogen receptor-negative, there is no need to avoid local therapies containing estrogen only. If you have tried the non-hormonal interventions discussed previously and have not found the symptom relief you need, contact a healthcare provider for a discussion about local estrogen therapy. Often, you will find that a gynecologist or a women's health practitioner is very skilled at helping you find the right combination of products to relieve vaginal and urinary symptoms.

It is helpful for breast cancer patients to remember that clinical studies show that the local delivery of estrogen is very low with both Vagifem® vaginal suppository tablets and the Estring® vaginal ring. Vaginal creams deliver a much higher amount of estrogen into the systemic circulation. Vagifem® and Estring® are better treatment choices for women concerned about the systemic absorption of estrogen.

Intravaginal DHEA Suppository

DHEA (dehydroepiandrosterone) is a natural hormone produced in the adrenal glands. DHEA leads to the production of androgens and estrogens. When formulated into a vaginal suppository, it can be inserted into the vagina to treat vaginal dryness. A clinical study of 216 postmenopausal women with moderate to severe symptoms of vaginal atrophy received vaginally-administered DHEA daily for 12 weeks. Study results revealed increased desire, increased arousal, increased orgasm and reduced pain during sexual activity. There was no reported increase of estrogen in blood levels, making DHEA an option for women who have had estrogen receptor-positive breast cancer. DHEA suppositories require a physician's prescription and can be prepared by a compounding pharmacist. Discuss this option with your physician.

Clinical studies on the synthetic DHEA suppository, Prasterone®, have been completed and the drug is awaiting FDA approval.

New Medication for Vaginal Dryness

Osphena® is a new non-estrogen pill taken to reduce painful intercourse caused by vaginal dryness due to menopause or chemotherapy treatment. Osphena® effectively treats vaginal dryness by restoring the tissues in the vaginal area. Because it works like estrogen in the lining of the uterus, it can slightly increase the risk of having uterine cancer, strokes and blood clots. These risks are similar to those of taking oral birth control pills.

Vaginal Dryness and Painful Intercourse

Damaged Vaginal Tissue Restoration

If you have experienced pain or bleeding after intercourse, it is recommended that you repair the damage that has occurred to the vaginal tissues. Repairing the damaged tissues requires a plan and interventions to allow the tissues to heal and return to a healthy condition before penetrative intercourse is attempted again. The goal is to heal the damaged tissues and to increase blood flow to the tissues.

Repairing damaged tissues caused by estrogen deficiency calls for a sexual partner's understanding. Before you begin the restoration plan outlined below, share this information with your partner. Assure your partner that your goal is to repair your vaginal tissues and then to keep them healthy by participating in frequent sexual encounters. Most partners are happy to participate when they understand the goal.

Steps to Vaginal Tissue Restoration:

- Stop any additional damage. Absolutely no vaginal friction should occur until tissues have completely healed.
- Repair the damaged skin and tissues by gently massaging internally and externally with Vitamin E daily to keep tissues moisturized.
  - Puncture a Vitamin E capsule, squeeze oil onto fingers, insert fingers into the vagina and apply using light pressure.
  - Next, apply to the external genital tissues using gentle pressure while massaging oil into tissues.
  - For extremely dry vaginal tissues, you can open several Vitamin E capsules and generously apply oil to a tampon and insert into the vagina for several hours.
  - Gradually increase the pressure of finger massage each day while applying the Vitamin E oil.
- After one or two weeks of Vitamin E application with massage, the next step is to increase the blood flow to the vagina, which will speed healing. This is accomplished through sexual arousal that brings increased blood flow to the genitals and vagina. Ask your partner to participate in sexual foreplay until you are fully aroused. Use a lubricant or coconut oil to reduce any friction. Gentle touching of the clitoris will promote sexual arousal. Aim for sexual arousal without penetration. The goal is to increase blood flow, which promotes continued healing of tissues.

Chapter 5

Tissues need to heal fully before penetration occurs.
- Attempt sexual arousal as often as possible to promote blood flow for one to two weeks. Continue daily massage of Vitamin E.
- When tissues are completely healed, usually in three to four weeks, you are ready to attempt penetration. Prepare by liberally applying a lubricant to both partners before penetration. Attempt penetration. If it is painful, stop immediately and revert to sexual arousal and Vitamin E massage for an additional week. Then, repeat the process of attempting penetration.
- After tissues are healed, regular, non-painful intercourse helps tissues remain healthy.

Vaginal Stenosis

Women who suffer from painful intercourse caused by vaginal dryness for an extended period of time often avoid penetrative intercourse to prevent pain. When they do attempt intercourse, they may find that they have developed a narrowing of the vaginal opening that makes penetration very unpleasant. This condition is called vaginal stenosis. If you experience this condition, consult a physician.

Vaginal stenosis requires treatment for dryness along with the usage of vaginal dilators to gradually stretch tissues back to the their original size. During an exam, your physician will measure your vagina to determine the appropriate size dilator to be used to begin stretching the tissues.

You will be instructed about the appropriate sizes of dilators and how to use them. Dilators are usually inserted 3 to 5 times a week in conjunction with vaginal exercises. When one size becomes easy to fully insert, a slightly larger size is then recommended. Gradually, the vaginal opening is stretched to its original size. Treatment for vaginal dryness is always an essential part of vaginal stenosis treatment. For additional vaginal stenosis information, refer to *Appendix B: Vaginal Dilator Therapy* on page 179.

Vaginal Dryness Precautions:
- Avoid vaginal douches, unless prescribed by a physician
- Avoid deodorant sprays, perfumes or powders applied to external genitals
- Avoid bubble baths or hot tubs

Vaginal Dryness and Painful Intercourse

- Avoid tight clothing
- Avoid synthetic fabrics in the crotch of panties
- Avoid panty liners containing deodorant
- Avoid tampons
- Avoid long-term use of antihistamines such as Benadryl® or Chlor-Trimeton®
- Avoid long-term use of decongestants such as Sudafed®

Seeking Medical Help

It is recommended that you request an appointment for an examination to look for any other causes that may be contributing to painful intercourse. Other conditions may include bacterial or fungal overgrowths, allergic reactions, trauma and benign or malignant tumors. A complete examination ensures that your recommended treatment is accurate and designed to meet your specific needs. During this appointment, the healthcare provider will discuss the risks and benefits of treatment.

When you visit a healthcare provider for vaginal dryness or painful intercourse, provide the following information about your history:

- Describe the problems you are experiencing: dryness, burning, itching, urinary urgency or frequency, urinary leakage, pain during penetrative intercourse, pain or bleeding after intercourse.
- How long you have experienced the problems.
- The interventions you have used to treat the problems and how successful they have been.

Chapter 5

Remember

- *Vaginal dryness, painful intercourse and urinary symptoms are side effects of low estrogen levels. Multiple interventions are available to alleviate these symptoms.*

- *Vaginal moisturizers help retain moisture in the vagina but are not designed as a lubricant for intercourse.*

- *Lubricants, applied liberally before intercourse, reduce the discomfort or pain from vaginal dryness. The selection of the best lubricant varies according to condom use, desire to become pregnant and sensitivity to glycerin or paraben.*

- *Some women find that moisturizers and lubricants do not adequately relieve their symptoms. Local estrogen therapy options, including vaginal creams, vaginal rings and vaginal tablets, may be needed to treat symptoms.*

- *Local estrogen therapy temporarily increases systemic estrogen levels, but the levels quickly fall and remain within menopausal levels, making it a safe therapy for estrogen receptor-positive breast cancer patients. Most patients experience a reduction of estrogen-deprivation symptoms within several weeks and adequate relief after 12 weeks. Local estrogen therapy requires a prescription from a healthcare professional.*

- *Women who have experienced severe pain or bleeding after intercourse find great benefit from a sexual restoration plan for damaged vaginal tissues. Vaginal restoration consists of daily Vitamin E vaginal massages throughout the program, then, after several weeks, sexual arousal without penetration is added to increase vaginal blood flow. The final step is intercourse with penetration.*

- *Vaginal stenosis is a narrowing of the estrogen-deprived vagina that prevents penetration. The treatment goal is to stretch the vaginal canal by using vaginal dilators inserted into the vagina.*

Chapter 6

Urinary Changes

Urinary problems are common to women after cancer treatment and menopause. Not only does the loss of estrogen cause changes in the vagina, it greatly impacts all the urinary tract lining cells. Lack of estrogen causes these cells to become thin and easily irritated, which causes a number of urinary changes to occur. Estrogen loss also causes the muscles in the bladder that control urinary flow to become lax, along with muscles that support your bladder, reducing the ability to hold or stop urine.

Common urinary problems after the loss of estrogen include increased frequency, burning after urination, increased infections, increased urgency and increased stress incontinence (leaking of urine). Women do not hesitate to seek a physician's help with a urinary tract infection, but often will not discuss urinary urgency or leaking of urine due to embarrassment. These are common and treatable medical conditions. It is important to discuss any changes in your urinary health with your physician. Getting help with these problems is part of your sexual restoration.

Common Urinary Problems

Frequency and Urgency

The first symptom most women notice is an increased need to urinate frequently. Frequent bathroom trips are required during the day, and nighttime urination may require getting up several times a night, which interrupts sleep. The next bothersome symptom is urinary urgency or the sudden need to urinate. Urgency causes a person to have to locate a toilet quickly after an urge to urinate occurs.

Urinary Incontinence

Urinary incontinence is the involuntary leakage of urine. Incontinence can be very embarrassing and often limits one's activities because of the fear of leaking urine. There are two types of urinary incontinence: urge incontinence and stress incontinence.

Chapter 6

- **Urge Incontinence** is the inability to hold urine in once an urge to urinate occurs. Getting to a nearby toilet becomes a challenge and if one is not located, leaking occurs.
- **Stress Incontinence** is when urine leaks after sneezing, coughing, laughing, heavy lifting, fast walking or running. Childbirth increases the potential for urinary problems because it weakens the bladder's supportive ligaments. Women who have lost the elasticity of the bladder muscles due to low estrogen levels, and have weakened bladder ligaments from childbirth, experience stress incontinence at a higher rate. Urine leakage may also occur during sexual intercourse, which causes embarrassment.

Treatment of Urinary Symptoms

The good news is that the medications to treat urinary symptoms caused by decreased estrogen are the same medications used to treat vaginal dryness. As discussed in the previous chapter, there are three types of local estrogen therapy used to treat urinary problems—vaginal creams (Premarin®, Estrace®, Estragyn®), vaginal rings (Estring® or Femring®) or vaginal tablets (Vagifem®). These are inserted into the vagina, and over a period of 8 to 12 weeks, the vaginal and urinary tissues are replenished and symptoms decrease greatly. In one study of local vaginal estrogen therapy, over 60 percent of patients had less pain during urination and experienced relief from sudden urinary urges after local estrogen therapy. See *Chapter 5: Vaginal Dryness and Painful Intercourse* for additional information about local estrogen therapy.

Incontinence Interventions and Treatment

The first interventions for stress incontinence are Kegel exercises and local vaginal estrogen. Performing Kegel exercises strengthens the pelvic floor muscles, while local vaginal estrogen restores the estrogen-deprived urinary cells. Most women find that these interventions bring a manageable degree of relief from their symptoms.

Urinary Changes

Kegel Exercises

Identifying the Correct Muscle

Determining the correct muscle to exercise is the first step to performing Kegel exercises. To identify your pelvic floor muscles, begin to urinate and then stop urination in midstream. The muscle used to stop urination is the muscle you will be exercising during Kegel exercises. Once you have identified the muscle, do not make a practice of contracting it to stop your urinary stream. Stopping the urine stream is done only to identify the muscle.

Performing Kegel Exercises:

- Empty your bladder.
- Lie flat on your back. (May also be done while sitting or standing.)
- Tighten the pelvic floor muscle that you have identified and hold tight for five seconds.
- Relax the muscle for five seconds.
- Repeat five times.
- Attempt to increase the time of holding the muscle tight to 10 seconds; then relaxing it for 10 seconds.
- Breathe normally during the exercise; avoid holding your breath.
- Repeat the exercise 3 times daily.

For women who do not get relief from these interventions, an appointment with a physician specializing in female urinary problems is the next step. An incontinence specialist may be a urologist or a urogynecologist (gynecologist specializing in urinary problems). An appointment with a specialist will determine which additional tests may be needed to identify your specific problem. Tests will determine whether you have stress incontinence, urge incontinence or both. After the testing, your healthcare provider will explain the best options for your condition.

Stress Incontinence Treatment

For stress incontinence that does not respond to Kegel exercises, surgery may be needed because weakened pelvic floor muscles have allowed the bladder neck and urethra to drop. Surgery seeks to lift the organs back into the correct position. After successful surgery, you are less likely to leak urine from the bladder when sneezing, coughing, laughing, walking, running fast, lifting heavy objects or during sexual intercourse.

Chapter 6

Several types of surgical procedures are performed for stress incontinence. After evaluating your condition, the doctor will discuss the available surgical options. The type of surgery selected depends on your preference, your health and your doctor's expertise.

Urge Incontinence Treatment

With urge incontinence, urine is leaked because the bladder muscles squeeze or contract at the wrong time. Often, these contractions occur no matter how much urine is in the bladder. You feel an urge to urinate and find that you are not able to control your urine until you get to a bathroom. Treatment for urge incontinence includes pelvic exercise, bladder training, lifestyle changes, medication and possibly surgery. Surgery is done much less often for urge incontinence than for stress incontinence.

Cystitis and Urinary Tract Infections

When estrogen levels are low, women may experience an increase in irritation of the tissues lining the inside of the bladder wall, called cystitis. Cystitis causes urinary frequency (more than eight times during the day; more than two times at night), urinary urgency and burning with urination. The inflammation of the tissues increases the risk of a urinary tract infection (UTI) if bacteria enters through your urethra and begins to multiply. The infection may then spread to include the kidneys and become a serious health condition, requiring an antibiotic.

Urinary Tract Infection Symptoms:

- Cloudy urine
- Pain or burning with urination
- Foul or strong odor
- Strong need to urinate often, even right after the bladder has been emptied
- Pressure or cramping in the lower abdomen or back
- Blood in urine (color of tea)
- Feeling tired and shaky
- Low-grade fever or chills accompanying other symptoms (a sign that the infection has reached your kidneys)

If you suspect a urinary tract infection, report it to your healthcare provider immediately. Symptoms will continue to worsen until it is treated. A urine

Urinary Changes

culture is usually performed, and antibiotic medication is prescribed for an infection. Medication to treat the discomfort and burning may also be prescribed. It is important that you continue to take all medication prescribed, even after symptoms disappear. It is also helpful to increase your water intake during an infection. The average recommendation to maintain water balance is eight 8-ounce glasses per day.

Tips To Deal With Urinary Changes

If you are dealing with urinary changes, the following tips may be helpful:

- Stay well-hydrated. Drink lots of water.
- Urinate often to prevent a sudden urge from a full bladder. Do not hold your urine for long periods of time.
- Limit coffee, tea, soda and alcoholic drinks which increase urgency.
- Limit liquids several hours before bedtime to reduce nighttime urination.
- Urinate after sexual intercourse to prevent bladder infections.
- Perform Kegel exercises.
- Wear a panty liner, if you are experiencing urinary leakage.
- Talk to your doctor about your urinary problems.
- Consider local estrogen replacement to treat both vaginal and urinary symptoms.
- Ask for a referral to a physician specializing in incontinence if problems remain after the above interventions.

Chapter 6

Remember

- Due to a lack of estrogen, urinary problems are common for menopausal and chemo-treated women. These problems are more common for women who have a history of vaginal childbirth.

- Urinary frequency, burning, increase in infections, urinary urgency or stress incontinence are all treatable urinary problems.

- Discuss your urinary problems with your physician. Ask for a referral to a urogynecologist or urologist if you are experiencing urinary incontinence.

- Incontinence testing by the urinary specialist will determine which type of incontinence you are experiencing and what options are best suited for your condition.

- Do not suffer in silence; there are answers and help available.

Chapter 7

Hot Flashes and Night Sweats

A hot flash is a recurring, sudden sensation of increased body heat that begins in one region of the body and spreads quickly to the face, neck and chest and lasts several minutes. Often, hot flashes are accompanied by palpitations (rapid, fluttering or pounding heart) or acute feelings of anxiety, followed by chills. Hot flashes are caused by irregular expansion and contraction of the small blood vessels, which is due to a lack of estrogen. They are unexpected and can be very bothersome. Hot flashes are associated with increased sweating and night sweats.

> **Patient Quote**
>
> "My one great wish at this time is that I can attend my son's wedding this August (9 months away) and not wet my dress during the wedding or reception from hot flashes and sweating. I have struggled with having 10 – 12 episodes a day for over two years. I haven't been able to sleep over 2 – 3 hours at a time during this time because of night sweats. My doctor says that many women have the same problem, and he offered no help. I am so discouraged. Is there any hope or help for me?"
>
> — EduCare Focus Group

Night sweats that occur while you are asleep will awaken you to find your pajamas and bed linens damp from perspiration. Night sweats are usually followed by an extreme feeling of coolness. Within minutes, you go from burning-up to chilly. In addition to these bothersome symptoms, the physical impact of sleep disturbance can be a significant quality-of-life issue. Sleep disturbances result in daytime fatigue.

The frequency of hot flashes varies from a few a day to as many as twenty a day.

Chapter 7

Hot Flash Frequency

Number of Hot Flashes Experienced Daily

Before Diagnosis:

Per Day: 0 ....81%
Per Day: 1-2 ....10%
Per Day: 3-5 ....8%
Per Day: 6-10 ....0%
Per Day: 10+ Per Day 0%

During Treatment:

Per Day: 0 ....32%
Per Day: 1-2 ....19%
Per Day: 3-5 ....25%
Per Day: 6-10 ....11%
Per Day: 10+ 13%

6 Months After Treatment:

Per Day: 0 ....12%
Per Day: 1-2 ....26%
Per Day: 3-5 ....32%
Per Day: 6-10 ....13%
Per Day: 10+ 17%

12 Months After Treatment:

Per Day: 0 ....14%
Per Day: 1-2 ....25%
Per Day: 3-5 ....27%
Per Day: 6-10 ....20%
Per Day: 10+ 14%

Hot flashes were reported to be one of the most troubling side effects of treatment, and progressively increased after treatment ended.

Night Sweat Frequency

Number of Night Sweats Experienced Daily

Before Diagnosis:

Per Day: 0 ....75%
Per Day: 1-2 ....22%
Per Day: 3-5 ....3%
Per Day: 6-10 ....0%
Per Day: 10+ Per Day 0%

During Treatment:

Per Day: 0 ....33%
Per Day: 1-2 ....25%
Per Day: 3-5 ....29%
Per Day: 6-10 ....9%
Per Day: 10+ 6%

6 Months After Treatment:

Per Day: 0 ....25%
Per Day: 1-2 ....28%
Per Day: 3-5 ....36%
Per Day: 6-10 ....7%
Per Day: 10+ 4%

12 Months After Treatment:

Per Day: 0 ....26%
Per Day: 1-2 ....42%
Per Day: 3-5 ....17%
Per Day: 6-10 ....9%
Per Day: 10+ 5%

Hot Flashes and Night Sweats

The changes experienced during a hot flash are not life-threatening, but they are quality-of-life threatening. For breast cancer patients whose cancer was estrogen receptor-positive and are currently taking tamoxifen or an aromatase inhibitor to reduce the risk of recurrence, the potential for hot flashes increases.

Hot Flash and Night Sweat Management

The first step in the management of hot flashes is learning how to control your environment to reduce their impact.

Tips for Dealing With Hot Flashes and Night Sweats:

- Look for a pattern. Expecting hot flashes can give you a sense of control and help you prepare. Some women experience hot flashes around the clock while others experience them during the nighttime hours. Determine your pattern of occurrence so that you can prepare.
- Dress in light, layered clothing so that you can remove outer garments when a hot flash occurs. Avoid turtlenecks. Wear slip-on shoes that can be quickly removed so that you can place your feet on the cold floor.
- Avoid hot environments like saunas, hot showers, hot tub baths, Jacuzzis, sunbathing or direct summer sun.
- Purchase small electric fans for your office, kitchen and bedroom.
- Drink cold drinks. Avoid hot drinks. When a hot flash starts, drink cold water to reduce the sensation and to keep hydrated.
- Avoid highly seasoned foods, alcohol and drinks with large amounts of caffeine (coffee, tea and soft drinks), which can stimulate hot flashes.
- Sleep in a cool room. Use cotton sheets and bed coverings that can be removed easily. Wear cotton pajamas.
- Avoid emotionally stimulating situations. Increased stress increases hot flash occurrences.
- Carry a small package of facial wet wipes to cool your skin when needed.

Hot Flash and Night Sweat Medications

The most frequently prescribed medications to reduce hot flashes for cancer patients are one of the SSRIs (selective serotonin reuptake inhibitors) or SNRIs (selective norepinephrine reuptake inhibitors). Citalopram (Celexa®), escitalopram (Lexapro®), venlafaxine (Effexor®, Pristiq®) and fluvoxamine (Luvox®) are most often prescribed. However, it is essential

Chapter 7

that you be aware that while these antidepressant medications reduce the frequency and sensation of hot flashes, they may also lower your sex drive. A clinical study published in the *Journal of Clinical Psychiatry* involving 6,297 patients taking an SSRI reported that 37 percent experienced sexual dysfunction as a side effect. This fact often creates a dilemma for patients when deciding which symptom is the most bothersome and which one needs treatment.

If your hot flashes are bothersome enough to require an SSRI or SNRI for control, you can take the medication and monitor your sexual response. Hopefully, you will be in the 63 percent of people who do not experience sexual side effects. If you do experience an inability to achieve orgasm, one tip you can try is to change the time of day you take your medication. If you most often engage in sexual activity in the evening, you can try taking your medication before going to sleep at night rather than in the morning. In the evenings, the amount of drug will be at the lowest level in the blood and cause the lowest level of sexual side effects.

Another suggestion to lower sexual side effects is to ask your doctor about decreasing the dosage of your medication to the lowest level required to control your hot flashes. Lowering the medication dosage will cause the least potential for sexual side effects.

Some women find that taking 50 mg of Benadryl®, an over-the-counter antihistamine, at night allows them to sleep through hot flashes.

Prescription Medication Alternatives

Other prescription medications that may offer hot flash relief for some women, without impacting sexual function are:

- **Gabapentin (Neurontin®, Gralise®, Horizant®, Gabarone®):** Gabapentin is an anti-seizure medication that has been moderately effective in reducing hot flashes. Side effects can include drowsiness, dizziness and headaches.
- **Paroxetine (Brisdelle®):** Paroxetine is the only FDA approved non-hormonal formula specifically for hot flashes.
- **Clonidine (Catapres®, Kapvay® and Others):** Clonidine, a pill or patch typically used to treat high blood pressure, may provide some relief from hot flashes. Side effects include dizziness, drowsiness, dry mouth and constipation.

Hot Flashes and Night Sweats

Talk to your healthcare provider about your hot flashes, and ask for a recommendation for symptom management. Do not continue to suffer. Seek help to reduce the impact on your quality of life.

Remember

- *Hot flashes are a side effect that most chemo-treated and menopausal women experience.*
- *Hot flashes and night sweats can rob you of your quality of life. If possible, you deserve interventions to help reduce their impact.*
- *First, try to control your environment to help reduce the frequency or intensity of your hot flashes.*
- *Ask your healthcare provider for recommendations. If an SSRI or SNRI medication is prescribed, monitor the sexual side effects you experience. If sexual side effects occur, try taking your medication at night (if your sexual encounters are usually at night) rather than in the morning. You may also consider lowering the dosage to the lowest level to control your hot flashes to determine if this helps decrease the impact on your sexual desire.*
- *If the sexual impact of SSRIs or SNRIs is high, ask for an alternative medication that does not have sexual side effects.*

Chapter 8

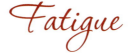

After cancer treatment, fatigue is the number one complaint of patients. Fatigue is a normal and expected side effect of cancer treatment. Fatigue is described as a sensation of exhaustion during or after normal activities, or a feeling of inadequate energy to begin these activities

What comes as a surprise to most cancer-treated women is that the fatigue does not end when treatment ends. The degree of fatigue experienced during cancer treatment decreases, but fatigue continues to linger for months or longer. Many side effects of treatment continue to contribute to fatigue.

Fatigue

- 62% experienced a decrease in energy **during** treatments
- 41% experienced a decrease in energy **six months after** treatment completion
- 22% experienced a decrease in energy **one year after** treatment completion

Returning to pretreatment energy levels was a gradual process with lingering fatigue persisting beyond one year after treatment conclusion.

— *EduCare Focus Group Data*

Suffering from fatigue drains the joy and enthusiasm out of life and leaves little room for an active, fulfilling sex life. Fatigue is a major saboteur of a couple's sex life. Restoring your sexuality requires identifying causes of fatigue and modifying or correcting them.

To restore your energy, it is necessary to look for any potential contributing causes of lingering fatigue. Sometimes, causes of fatigue after treatment may not be easily identified. In the following chapters, we will look at common causes that promote lingering fatigue. Some causes are obvious, but, some are often not suspected as being a contributing factor to fatigue.

Chapter 8

Physical Disorders Causing Fatigue

The first place to begin to search is with your current medical condition. Listed below are common physical disorders that directly cause fatigue as a side effect. These underlying disorders are identified through blood studies. This requires a physical evaluation by your physician. Without correction of these underlying medical conditions, your fatigue will linger.

- Iron deficiency with or without anemia
- Vitamin B12 deficiency
- Vitamin D deficiency
- Diabetes
- Hypothyroidism (low thyroid levels)

Ask your physician if your blood levels for each of the following are within normal range. These conditions can all be easily managed or corrected with supplements or medications.

Identifying Contributing Causes of Fatigue

After you rule out any physical disorder causing fatigue, exploring other potential contributing factors is necessary. Common fatigue-promoting causes are depression, anxiety and sleep problems. In the following chapters, we will explore these causes of fatigue and explain what you can do to correct or minimize the problems. We will then discuss how you can reduce fatigue through regular appropriate exercise and nutrition.

Fatigue is like a flashing yellow light on our car's dashboard. It warns us that there is something causing a problem that needs to be addressed.

Fatigue

Remember

- *Fatigue robs you of your energy to participate in may of life's daily activities.*

- *Fatigue is the number one side effect of treatment. It is an expected side effect that decreases at the end of treatment, but has a lingering effect. Fatigue levels should gradually decline during the months following treatment.*

- *Fatigue that does not decrease requires a close assessment of all contributing factors to rule out physical disorders of anemia, Vitamin B-12 deficiency, Vitamin D deficiency, diabetes and hypothyroid. These disorders, unless corrected, can sabotage efforts to regain your energy.*

- *Fatigue is like the flashing yellow light on the car dashboard. It is an indicator that something is causing a problem that needs attention.*

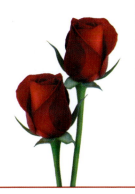

Chapter 9

Sleep Problems

The National Sleep Foundation reports that 48 percent of menopausal women experience sleep problems. Many women suffer from insomnia, which causes difficulty falling asleep, staying asleep or waking early. Insomnia causes fatigue the following day.

Insomnia can stem from unaddressed treatment for anxiety, depression or physical pain. Hot flashes or night sweats can also interrupt sleep. Sleep disturbances translate into fatigue the following day, which is often accompanied by irritability or anxiety. Suffering from disturbed sleep or insomnia no doubt puts a serious damper on the motivation and energy needed for sexual activity.

Fatigue plays a major role in sexual dysfunction. Taking steps to correct anything that contributes to fatigue is essential. Suffering from sleep deprivation is a major fatigue-contributing problem that needs attention if you want to get your sexual energy back.

Insomnia
- 91% increase in insomnia **during** treatment
- 73% increase in insomnia **six months after** treatment completion
- 61% increase in insomnia **one year after** treatment completion

The degree of insomnia correlated closely with the number of hot flashes and night sweats experienced by the patient.

— *EduCare Focus Group Data*

Addressing the issue of insomnia is an important component of reducing fatigue. It is helpful to understand factors that contribute to insomnia and learn how you can minimize their influence on your sleep.

Tips for Getting a Good Night's Sleep:
- Go to bed and get up at the same time each day to create a sleep pattern.

Chapter 9

- Exercise daily, but avoid strenuous exercise several hours before bedtime.
- Avoid daytime naps.
- Maintain the same sleep schedule on weekends. Avoid sleeping late.
- Establish a relaxing bedtime ritual such as a warm bath or reading.
- Avoid bright lights and working on a computer, tablet or phone a couple of hours before bedtime. Bright lights stimulate the brain. The blue wavelengths produced by your smartphone and other gadgets, such as energy-efficient LED light bulbs, significantly suppresses the production of melatonin, the hormone that makes you sleepy. Light-emitting devices engage and stimulate the mind, resulting in poor sleep. Cover LED lights on clocks, phones and computers in your bedroom to block the light.
- Keep the bedroom cool. Room temperature between 60 to 67 degrees is ideal for sleeping.
- Eliminate light in the bedroom that could disturb your sleep. Consider using blackout curtains, or eye shades.
- Eliminate any outside noise with earplugs, white noise machines, humidifiers, fans and other devices.
- Avoid caffeine 6 hours before bedtime. Remember, caffeine is found in many foods and drinks.
- Avoid eating a big meal 2 to 3 hours before bedtime. A high-protein snack such as yogurt eaten at bedtime, however, may help you to sleep longer.
- Avoid alcohol as a sleep promoter. Alcohol may cause you to fall asleep, but it robs you of REM and the deeper stages of sleep, which are the stages that make you feel most rested the next day.
- Wind down before bedtime by avoiding anxiety-provoking television shows. Instead, listen to calming music and drink a cup of chamomile tea to help you relax.
- Soak in a magnesium bath (one cup of Epsom salts added to warm bath water), which helps relax the body and can promote sleep.
- Sprinkle four or five drops of aromatherapy oils on a cotton ball or tissue and hold it close to your nose. Take 10 to 15 deep breaths. Lavender oil is known to be the best for promoting sleep.
- Rub magnesium oil on the back of the knees to promote relaxation. This oil can be found in health food stores or can be ordered online.

Sleep Problems

- Keep a sleep diary and record your sleeping habits and awakenings to find common patterns. Record any identified causes such as hot flashes, night sweats, pain, activity or caffeinated drinks. These records are helpful for a healthcare provider to determine interventions to promote sleep.

Insomnia Medications

Benadryl® (diphenhydramine) is an over-the-counter antihistamine medication that causes relaxation and drowsiness. Benadryl® contains the same medication that is added to Tylenol PM® and Aleve PM® to make them nighttime medications. Some people find that 50 mg of Benadryl® taken at bedtime will allow about four hours of uninterrupted sleep. Benadryl® is a safe alternative to prescription sleep medication. The medication can be purchased in tablet or liquid form. *Precaution: Benadryl® will increase vaginal dryness if used daily.*

If you identify anything that is awakening you when you keep your sleep diary, discuss this with a healthcare provider. Alleviating pain or hot flashes may be the answer to reducing your insomnia.

Prescription sleep medication is helpful for short-term use. Most prescription sleep medication is habit-forming and can be difficult to stop when used for longer periods of time than recommended.

Snoring and Sleep Apnea

You may be surprised to find the topic of snoring in a book about sexuality. However, snoring can be a hidden source of fatigue. Fatigue is a side effect of snoring and sleep apnea (periods of no breathing). Traditionally, snoring has been attributed to males, but newer data shows the ratio between male and female snorers to be 2:1, with women snoring less loudly than men. Women often do not realize that they snore. However, if they do know they snore, they may not realize that it is a health threat and a cause of their daytime fatigue. Often, women are too embarrassed to report their snoring to a physician,

Why Women Snore

Snoring is caused when the flow of air from the mouth or nose is blocked, which makes the tissues of the airway vibrate. This blockage may be from a narrowing in the nose, mouth or throat. When we lie on our backs,

Chapter 9

gravity pulls the palate, tonsils and tongue backward. This often narrows the airway enough to cause a disturbance in airflow, tissue vibration and snoring. Most snoring in women occurs after menopause (or chemopause) when estrogen levels decrease, which causes the elasticity of all body tissues to decrease greatly. The lack of tissue elasticity allows the airway tissues to sag and block the airway, which is a frequent cause of snoring.

If you are a habitual snorer, you impair your sleep quality and increase your risk for obstructive sleep apnea. Sleep apnea can occur in both people who snore and people who do not snore. Sleep apnea is defined as periods of not breathing for 10 seconds or more. The interruption is caused by a partial obstruction of the airway. When these periods of not breathing occur, you receive inadequate levels of oxygen to the body. These interruptions cause frequent waking from sleep even though you are not aware of it. When these awakenings occur, more time is spent in light sleep than in restorative, deeper sleep. Most people do not realize that they have sleep apnea. After being in bed for eight hours, you assume you are getting enough sleep and wonder why you feel so tired the next day. If you are experiencing sleep apnea, you are sleep-deprived. Sleep deprivation leads to fatigue, and fatigue leads to less energy for an active life, including sex.

The symptoms of snoring and sleep apnea have an adverse effect on neurological and psychological function. Snoring and sleep apnea cause brain fog, which creates difficulty concentrating, memory impairment and translates into poor work performance. Symptoms such as daytime fatigue, headaches, insomnia, tension and depression are also increased in snorers with sleep apnea. Unaware that they are snoring, women usually only report symptoms of insomnia and depression to their doctors. Even if these symptoms are treated, they do not correct the underlying problem of oxygen deprivation from sleep apnea. Reporting snoring is necessary so that you can receive help.

Ask your partner if you snore. If you do, ask your partner to observe your breathing while you sleep to see if you have periods when you appear to stop breathing for a short time. If the answer is yes, it will be beneficial to have this checked by a sleep specialist. Sleep studies can determine how often you stop breathing and the impact this is having on your sleep.

Sleep Problems

Correcting sleep apnea is essential to increasing your energy during the day. Once identified, there are many causes of sleep apnea that can be easily corrected.

Symptoms That Need Evaluation:
- You snore loudly enough to disturb the sleep of others or yourself.
- You experience shortness of breath, which awakens you from sleep.
- You have intermittent pauses in your breathing during sleep.
- You have excessive daytime drowsiness that causes you to fall asleep easily while reading, watching television, riding as a passenger in a car or even working.

Treatments for Snoring or Sleep Apnea:
- **Dental Devices:** Dental devices are custom-made by a dentist to address your specific problem. These devices have proven effective in reducing snoring and can be useful in correcting mild to moderate cases of obstructive sleep apnea.
- **Nasal Devices:** For people with narrow nasal passages, snoring can be alleviated with a nasal device. Nasal strips open the anterior nasal valve (front part of the nose). If this is the main, or only, area of narrowing, snoring may improve with the use of these strips, but this is frequently not the case.
- **Medications:** Some people only snore when they have colds or allergies. Nasal steroid sprays and nasal decongestants may be used to improve nasal breathing. These are very helpful in treating minor allergies or irritation. Steroid sprays decrease inflammation in the nasal passages. Very little of the steroid is absorbed into the body, so there are few side effects with these sprays. Nasal decongestants that shrink the blood vessels in the nose can also be used to improve snoring caused by nasal congestion. *Precaution: It is necessary to use as directed on the label. When used excessively, nasal sprays may cause localized swelling.*
- **Nasal CPAP (Continuous Positive Airway Pressure):** A device that is commonly used in patients after a sleep study shows obstructive sleep apnea. This device works by providing continuous, increased air pressure to prevent airway narrowing during breathing. A mask that is connected by tubing to a pump that keeps the pressure of the inspired air at a higher than normal level is worn at night while sleeping.

Chapter 9

- **Surgery:** Surgery is an option only after a formal sleep study (polysomnogram) confirms that snoring is not a symptom of obstructive sleep apnea. If sleep apnea is the case, CPAP needs to be prescribed and attempted as the first step. Surgery is an option to reduce snoring if it is caused by an obstruction or narrowing of the airway that can be surgically corrected.

If you are a snorer and suffer from fatigue, insomnia or both from frequent awakenings during the night, seek an evaluation from a professional.

Remember

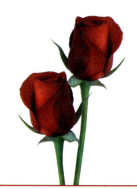

- *Insomnia or sleep interruption is a significant contributor to fatigue. Fatigue is a major blocker of sexual desire. Restoring normal sexual function requires you to evaluate possible sleep disrupters.*

- *If you are experiencing hot flashes or night sweats which awaken you during the night, contact your physician.*

- *Snoring or sleep apnea can greatly contribute to not getting adequate sleep. Have your partner monitor your sleep to determine whether you snore and whether you have brief periods of sleep apnea. If so, contact a sleep specialist to determine the degree of your condition.*

Chapter 10

Depression and Anxiety

Often, books on sexuality jump straight to interventions and techniques to ramp up the sex drive without discussing the most common causes of dysfunction after cancer treatment—depression or anxiety. Without a doubt, having a sexual rendezvous is not on a patient's list of desired activities if she is experiencing depression. Depression robs an individual of the energy and desire to participate in daily activities, including sex. If you desire to get your sex life back on track, it is essential to determine whether depression or anxiety are contributing factors to your lack of desire.

Mood Swings

Mood swings are an extreme or rapid change in one's mood. From happy to sad. From peaceful to angry. From laughing to crying. Extreme mood changes have a direct impact and can sabotage a person's relationships with others and their own personal happiness if not managed.

Wide swings in hormonal balance can create mood swings. During the focus groups, patients were asked about their changes in mood during and after treatment.

Mood Swings
56% increase in mood swings **during** treatment
44% increase in mood swings **six months after** treatment completion
22% increase in mood swings **one year after** treatment completion
— EduCare Focus Group Data

When a woman goes through chemotherapy and her hormonal balance changes, mood swings are a common manifestation. When mood swings are coupled with the continuous stress of treatment, anxiety or depression may occur. The gradual changes that anxiety or depression bring are

Chapter 10

subtle and may not be recognized by the patient. The patient may consider the symptoms she is feeling to be a normal part of having cancer and undergoing cancer treatment. Therefore, the symptoms of anxiety or depression may go unaddressed.

Anxiety and depression are serious sabatogers of a person's mental and physical health and are a roadblock to reestablishing a vibrant, healthy sexual relationship. They can have severe consequences on recovery by decreasing physical stamina and decreasing immunity. Depression and anxiety have effective treatments available to control or eliminate their impact. However, the symptoms must be recognized, reported and treated. If you find yourself struggling with your emotions, you are not alone. Members of the focus group experienced a common struggle.

Depression Episodes

- 129% increase in depressive episodes **during** treatment
- 96% increase in depressive episodes **six months after** treatment completion
- 75% increase in depressive episodes **one year after** treatment completion

Episodes of short-term depression (not clinical depression) increased greatly during treatment and remained a lingering problem after treatment completion.

— *EduCare Focus Group Data*

The purpose of this chapter is to help you recognize the symptoms of depression and anxiety, and to let you know how to seek help. As you read through the symptoms for each, determine if you share the same feelings, and if so, reach out for help.

Understanding Depression

Depression is more than just feeling down or feeling blue for a short period after a loss or disappointment. It is a serious condition with symptoms that affect both the mind and the body. It also has a major effect on sexual functioning. The first step to distinguishing the difference between feeling blue or experiencing depression is to understand the characteristics of each. Feeling blue means you feel sad, but you can still enjoy parts of your life, such as a family gathering, a movie or seeing a friend. Depression, however, causes an individual to find it difficult to enjoy any area of her life. A depressed person is unable to find joy in anything.

Depression and Anxiety

Depression Symptoms:
(Check the symptoms you may be experiencing.)

- ☐ Continuous feelings of sadness
- ☐ Social withdrawal from friends or family
- ☐ Feelings of worthlessness
- ☐ Feelings of hopelessness
- ☐ Excessive feelings of guilt
- ☐ Excessive fear of the future
- ☐ Slowed physical movement or speech
- ☐ Constant jitters or nervousness
- ☐ Low energy level; may feel tired all of the time
- ☐ Inability to make decisions
- ☐ Irrational thinking
- ☐ Constant anger or mistrust
- ☐ Obsessions about health and cancer recurrence
- ☐ Disinterest in food, or eating excessively
- ☐ Disinterest in work or day-to-day activities
- ☐ Disinterest in intimacy or sex
- ☐ Insomnia (difficulty falling asleep or staying asleep; waking early)
- ☐ Hypersomnia (sleeping too much)
- ☐ Frequent thoughts of death; thoughts that life is not worth living *(Please seek help from your healthcare team immediately.)*

If you have exhibited several of the listed symptoms for two weeks or longer, you need to reach out for help. Contact your physician. The encouraging fact is that depression usually responds positively to a combination of counseling and medication. Depression may be treated with counseling to identify and strengthen coping skills. Mental health counselors are trained to help people identify how they respond to their environments and what they can do to improve their coping skills. Antidepressant medications are designed to change the body chemistry in order to promote a better mood. Diet and exercise have also been proven to be beneficial to reduce depression and stress.

Depression is not a sign of weakness. It is a legitimate condition that is experienced by many people after a major crisis or loss. Most depression is time-limited; thus, short-term counseling and medication will help during this period of adjustment. Identifying symptoms and seeking help are the first steps to resolving depression. If you feel that this may be occurring in your life, call your healthcare provider for the help available to overcome your depression.

Chapter 10

Understanding Anxiety

Webster's dictionary defines anxiety as, *"A state of uneasiness, apprehension, uncertainty and fear resulting from the anticipation of a realistic or fantasized threatening event or situation, often impairing physical and psychological functioning."* Anxiety, like depression, takes control of one's emotions.

Anxiety is a normal first reaction when an event presents a real danger or threat. The anxiety occurs because of a person's perception of her inability to control or change the threat in her life. Anxiety can also occur when a person views a situation as threatening to her well-being. If anxiety lingers long after the initial threat is over, it may become chronic anxiety.

Webster's dictionary describes chronic anxiety as, *"The feelings of a persistent, troubled state of mind, distress, and mental uneasiness."* Simply thinking about the situation creates feelings of apprehension and fear—you feel threatened. Chronic anxiety by itself is not a disease or illness, but can turn into a "disorder" when it interferes with a normal lifestyle.

Many people consider chronic anxiety, or a highly anxious state, to be normal: *"I've always been a nervous worrier."* They do not understand how chronic anxiety can affect the body. Eventually, chronic anxiety translates into physical illness because of the stress it places on the body. It is a condition that needs to be addressed for a full recovery to occur. For chronic anxiety, counseling is used to identify the coping skills needed to manage anxiety. Medication is also available. Chronic anxiety is not a condition you have to live with. Reach out to your healthcare provider and describe the symptoms you are experiencing.

Anxiety Symptoms:

(Check the symptoms you may be experiencing.)

- ☐ Nervous or edgy
- ☐ Apprehensive about the future
- ☐ Feeling powerless
- ☐ A sense of impending danger, panic or doom
- ☐ Increased heart rate
- ☐ Rapid breathing
- ☐ Sweating
- ☐ Trembling
- ☐ Difficulty thinking about anything other than present worry

Depression and Anxiety

Anxiety
- 88% increase in anxiety **during** treatment
- 52% increase in anxiety **six months after** treatment completion
- 33% increase in anxiety **one year after** treatment completion

— *EduCare Focus Group Data*

How to Determine Which You Are Experiencing

It may be difficult to determine which you are experiencing. Is it anxiety, or is it depression? The assessment below will help determine if you have mostly depression, mostly anxiety or a combination of both. Determining this will be helpful when you seek treatment from a healthcare professional.

Anxiety or Depression Assessment

Set 1

1. Do you feel nervous or edgy most of the day for no reason? .... YES NO
2. Do you sometimes panic when something happens? .... YES NO
3. Do you often feel scared, as if something bad is going to happen? .... YES NO
4. Are you sometimes too nervous to do anything? .... YES NO
5. Do you constantly feel stressed out? .... YES NO

                                                  TOTAL ___ ___

Set 2

1. Do you no longer feel confident in yourself to handle problems? .... YES NO
2. Do you feel hopeless about what is happening in your life? .... YES NO
3. Do you feel helpless about what is happening in your life? .... YES NO
4. Do you feel worthless as a person? .... YES NO
5. Do you sometimes think that life is not worth living? .... YES NO

                                                  TOTAL ___ ___

CHAPTER 10

Anxiety or Depression Assessment Scoring

Assessment Score

Total up the **YES** and **NO** answers to each set of questions:

- If you answered YES to more of the questions in Set 1, you may be experiencing anxiety.
- If you answered YES to more of the questions in Set 2, you may be experiencing depression.
- If you answered YES to more than three in each set, you may be experiencing both depression and anxiety.

Discuss this questionnaire with your physician or someone on your healthcare team. This guide can help you ask for the correct interventions.

Treatments for Depression or Anxiety

It is essential to know that both chronic depression and chronic anxiety can be treated successfully. Both are treated with a combination of learning personal coping skills by seeking professional counseling and drug therapy.

Professional Counseling

In some cases, professional counseling may be all that is needed. Counseling identifies weaknesses in coping skills and works to strengthen them. Often, talking to an understanding person accomplishes a lot for a depressed or anxious person. Counseling therapy, often called talk therapy or psychotherapy, allows a person to talk about past and present experiences, relationships, feelings, thoughts and behaviors that may be contributing to the problem. The counselor's aim is to identify major causes of stress and then help determine the best approach to solving the problems.

Medications

Medications may be needed to assist with the therapeutic process. These require a prescription from a physician or an advanced care practitioner. Some people feel there is a stigma to taking anti-anxiety or antidepressant medications. However, taking medications for depression or anxiety is no different than taking medication for diabetes. Diabetes or anxiety/depression are all uninvited and attack the body's functions. The good news is that each of these conditions can be successfully managed with

Depression and Anxiety

medications. Denying yourself medication to help with your acute anxiety or depression is like denying yourself insulin to treat diabetes.

Anti-Anxiety Medication

Anti-anxiety medications (benzodiazepines) are used to calm your nerves and agitation. Many women diagnosed with acute anxiety find that taking an anti-anxiety medication allows them to regain their composure, concentrate easier and sleep much better. When taken correctly, symptoms of anxiety are reduced within 30 – 90 minutes. If you are experiencing a high level of anxiety, do not hesitate to ask your physician for help. Medication will allow you to get the rest you need and make decisions in a timelier, more informed manner.

A doctor will usually prescribe these medications only for a short time to help you get through a particularly rough period of anxiety. Long-term anxiety is better controlled with other medications. Anti-anxiety medications for acute anxiety may be prescribed on a regular schedule or to be taken as needed during periods of high anxiety. Do not drive while taking these medications because they cause drowsiness. Remember, your healthcare team cannot know what you are experiencing or what you need if you don't tell them.

Medications for Anxiety

- Alprazolam (Xanax®)
- Lorazepam (Ativan®)
- Chlordiazepoxide (Librium®)
- Clonazepam (Klonopin®)
- Diazepam (Valium®)

Antidepressant Medications

Antidepressants are often prescribed to stabilize your mood. Unlike short-term anti-anxiety medications, which work immediately, antidepressants will take approximately two to three weeks to become effective. There are a number of antidepressant categories to treat depression. The categories most often prescribed are SSRIs (selective serotonin reuptake inhibitors) and SNRIs (serotonin–norepinephrine reuptake inhibitors). Both categories of medication treat depression symptoms by altering the balance of brain neurotransmitters.

Chapter 10

Prescribing antidepressant medication is not a one-size-fits-all approach. Both the medications and the dosages must be carefully matched to a patient's symptoms and overall health. Physicians must consider a number of factors. For example, if you are experiencing depression accompanied by fatigue, an SSRI will help with the fatigue, and some SSRIs will reduce hot flashes. The SSRIs are the most commonly prescribed group of antidepressants. Remind your physician if you are taking tamoxifen because some SSRIs have been shown to reduce its effectiveness.

Although SSRI and SNRI medications are effective in improving depression or anxiety, they may cause sexual side effects that include diminished sexual desire, trouble achieving and maintaining arousal, and difficulty achieving orgasm. The medications in this category include fluoxetine (Prozac®), sertraline (Zoloft®), paroxetine (Paxil®), citalopram (Celexa®) and venlafaxine (Effexor®).

There is an alternative medication that does not reduce sex drive. Bupropion (Wellbutrin®) treats depression while increasing sex drive and arousal in most women. This medication may be used in women who do not have anxiety along with their depression. Patients who are taking Wellbutrin® have reported symptom improvement within 4 – 8 weeks of treatment. Duloxetine (Cymbalta®) is also less likely to cause sexual dysfunction. Newer medications are also being developed.

It is important to understand that not all antidepressants are effective in all people. It may take several attempts before your physician finds the most effective medication for your needs. Remember, it takes time for the antidepressant medication to build up in your body before you feel the full effect. For this reason, it is important to contact your physician when you first recognize symptoms of depression.

Antidepressants are usually prescribed for an extended period and are withdrawn gradually when you and your physician feel you are ready. They need to be taken as prescribed, without skipping doses or stopping when symptoms are controlled. Anti-anxiety medication and an antidepressant may initially be prescribed at the same time. When the antidepressant begins to take effect, the anti-anxiety medication is often reduced, discontinued or used only when needed. Talk to your healthcare

Depression and Anxiety

team about the help you need to regain control of your emotions and improve the quality of your life.

Medications for Depression
■ Bupropion (Wellbutrin®) ■ Fluoxetine (Prozac®, Prozac Weekly®) ■ Citalopram (Celexa®) ■ Fluvoxamine (Luvox®) ■ Desvenlafaxine (Pristiq®) ■ Paroxetine (Paxil®, Paxil CR®, Pexeva®) ■ Duloxetine (Cymbalta®) ■ Sertraline (Zoloft®) ■ Escitalopram (Lexapro®) ■ Venlafaxine (Effexor®)

Strategy for Dealing With Antidepressant Sexual Side Effects

Often, cancer-treated women struggle with the decision of whether or not to take medication to treat their depression and/or hot flashes because of the potential impact on their sex drive. *"What should I do?"* is a common question women ask. In my experience with patients, it is necessary to correct the problem of depression and/or hot flashes because they can greatly impact your quality of life. Once you have control of your depression and/or hot flashes, then you can implement a strategy to find a balance between controlling your symptoms and maintaining your sexual desire.

Strategies to Manage Antidepressant Sexual Side Effects:

- **Wait-and-See Approach:** Not all women respond to medication with a decrease in sexual functioning. Some women find that the relief from the hot flashes, night sweats, insomnia and depression gives them renewed energy and even an interest in pursuing sexual activity. Wait to see what impact the antidepressant has on your quality of life. Usually, it takes at least a month or longer to fully evaluate your response to the medication.
- **Modify Medication Schedule:** If your sexual activity is usually in the evening, try taking the medication at bedtime rather than in the morning. The drug level will be at the lowest in the evening.
- **Dosage Decrease:** If you have sexual side effects after several months, talk to your doctor about reducing the medication dosage. Be aware that medication reduction may cause your primary complaints to return. Only after trying will you know if you can tolerate a lower dose.

Chapter 10

- **Drug Holiday:** Another strategy is to talk to your doctor about a drug holiday. This drug holiday would allow you to skip your medication for one to three days. During this time, you may experience an increase in desire. Some SSRI medications remain in your system too long for this to be an effective strategy. Your doctor will be aware if your medication falls into this category.
- **Medication Change:** Talk to your doctor about changing your medication to one that may have fewer sexual side effects.
- **Add a Medication:** Talk to your doctor about medications that can potentially be added to your antidepressant to reduce the sexual side effects. Drugs that have been successfully used for this include:
  - Amantadine (Symmetrel®)
  - Dextroamphetamine (Dexedrine®)
  - Methylphenidate (Ritalin®)
  - Pemoline (Cylert®)
  - Cyproheptadine (Periactin®)
  - Buspirone (BuSpar®)
  - Granisetron (Kytril®)

Guarding Your Future Sexuality

Getting help to reduce your anxiety or depression symptoms without impairing your future sexual functioning requires careful evaluation by a healthcare professional.

If you are suffering from either depression or anxiety, contact your healthcare provider for help. I suggest including a professional counselor along with a medical doctor. Counselors are skilled at identifying behaviors and thought patterns that may be contributing to your symptoms. A psychiatrist is a good choice because psychiatrists are both a medical doctor and a counselor. A psychiatrist can assess your symptoms and prescribe medications that are the most appropriate for you while keeping the preservation of your sexual desire as a goal. To get your sex life back on track, it is essential to address your depression or anxiety.

DEPRESSION AND ANXIETY

Remember

- *Depression and anxiety are common side effects of a cancer diagnosis and cancer treatment. It is essential to determine whether you are dealing with either anxiety or depression or both and to receive appropriate treatments to return to optimal sexual functioning.*

- *Depression and anxiety are not signs of personal weakness, but a response experienced by many women after a major stressor. Everyone will agree that cancer is a major stressor.*

- *Depression or anxiety can be treated successfully with medication. Professional counseling is helpful to identify coping skills and regain control of your life.*

- *Seek help from a professional who is aware of your desire for the treatment of depression and/or anxiety while preserving your sex drive.*

Chapter 11

Value of Exercise

Patients often ask, *"Why should I exercise when I am already so tired?"* People who have not participated in regular exercise may think of exercise as an additional activity that will decrease their available energy. If you recently completed cancer treatment, you are probably experiencing lingering fatigue. The idea of exercising when you are tired may seem absurd. In the past, the traditional recommendation was that when you are tired, "you need to rest," and many patients reverted to bed rest to manage their fatigue. It was believed that the more you rested, the more quickly you would recover. In reality, the opposite has been found to be true. Physical exercise restores energy and is a component of developing good physical health.

Studies have proven that too much rest can promote physiological changes that increase, rather than decrease, fatigue. Too much rest can actually decrease your energy.

The *"Fatigue in Cancer: A Multi-dimensional Approach"* study by Greenleaf and Kozlowski revealed, *"Maintenance of optimal health in a person requires a proper balance between exercise, rest and sleep, as well as time in an upright position."*

Rest Versus Activity Study Revealed:
- Too much rest promotes fatigue (creates an imbalance).
- Too little exercise promotes fatigue (creates an imbalance).
- A dynamic balance between rest and activity decreases fatigue.
- The conclusion was that people need to remain as active as possible during physical recovery. There must be a balance of activity and rest for maximum energy to be maintained.

Chapter 11

Clinical Study of 100 Cancer Patients Reveals Benefits of Exercise:
- Functioned as a stress relief mechanism in coping
- Increase in feeling of control over their lives
- Increase in measurable functional energy using peak oxygen uptake as an indicator of functional capacity
- Increase in internal control (ability to make decisions)
- Increase in mood elevation
- Decrease in tension and anxiety
- No harmful or debilitating effects reported
- Increase of 40 percent in functional capacity at end of 10 weeks

Another interesting outcome involved those who did not participate in regular exercise. Unlike those who exercised, those who did not participate reported a worsening of mood states. It is important that you understand the newer concepts of energy building, especially after a cancer diagnosis and treatment.

Rest Recommendations Based on the New Facts:
- Too much rest can decrease available energy.
- Exercise can build energy.
- Decreased movement may make a person feel worse.
- Excessive rest and inactivity are enemies of recovery.
- Too much rest can cause increased fatigue.
- Exercise and rest must be balanced to maintain or build energy.
- Maintaining or starting a moderate exercise program based on your present ability can speed your recovery after treatment and reduce lingering treatment symptoms. Exercise will not harm you.

Whatever exercise program you select and follow consistently will raise your energy levels and speed your psychological recovery by decreasing anxiety and depression. In addition, exercise reduces pain by promoting the release of natural painkillers, referred to as endorphins or natural morphine, into the body. There is a lot of benefit to gain from something that only requires time.

Value of Exercise

Lymphatic System: The Body's Waste Removal System

One of the greatest values of exercise is the removal of body waste from the cells into the lymphatic system. The lymphatic system is a network of vessels that are located in the circulatory system. The primary function of the lymphatic system is to transport a clear, colorless fluid containing white blood cells to pick up cellular waste and rid it of body toxins and other unwanted material by filtering it through lymph nodes. Lymph nodes are filtering chambers that contain white blood cells and act as the first level of defense against infection. There are 600 to 700 lymph nodes in the human body that filter the lymph fluid before it returns to the circulatory system. The tonsils, adenoids, spleen and thymus are all part of the lymphatic system.

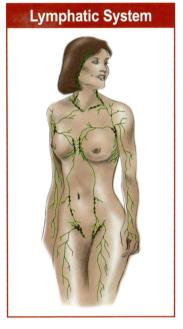

Lymphatic System

The lymphatic fluid flows in only one direction. This is unlike the blood system, which flows throughout the body in a continuous loop with valves to control the flow. The lymphatic system flows upward toward the neck in a system that has **no** valves. The fluid then enters into one of two subclavian veins located on either side of the neck near the collarbone, where the filtered fluid enters the blood. This means that lymph fluid **only** moves when adequate muscular pressure is placed around the vessels to push the fluid through the lymphatic system. This is the connection that is essential to understand with future immunity. Exercise increases the movement of lymph fluid in your body. The more your body moves, the more effectively the lymphatic system works to remove toxins from your body. Exercise is one of the major keys to increased immunity and restoring your energy.

Exercise Selection

Before beginning an exercise program, ask your physician if you have any limitations. Checking with your physician will allow you to select an exercise suitable to your present state of health. The goal is to select an exercise activity that you enjoy. Look at the time you set aside to participate

Chapter 11

in physical activity as a special time to take care of your health needs. The rewards will include increased physical stamina and psychological well-being.

What Type of Exercise Program Is Best?
The first step is to decide what type of physical activity is suitable for you and take steps to start. The right exercise for you is something you can physically do, you have the time to do, is convenient for you and you enjoy. Walking, Pilates, yoga, biking, swimming or gardening are all good choices.

You do not need to join a gym or health club to get adequate exercise unless you prefer exercising in this type of environment. You choose what works best for you. Some women prefer group exercise, while others prefer to exercise alone or with a family member or friend. If you consider participating in group exercise, a gym is an excellent place to receive the input of a trained specialist who can help you learn new types of exercise. Most gyms offer group classes and personal trainers. You can set your own pace, from slow and gentle to high cardio, according to your desire. Exercising at a gym is a great choice because weather does not interfere and they are usually open from early morning until late at night. If you have hesitations about going to a gym because you have not exercised in years and you are out of shape, STOP this thinking. This is the purpose of a gym. Everyone has a first day. I encourage you to visit a gym and discover what they have to offer. Most gyms offer a free pass for several days or a week to enable you to explore the option with no commitment. Many gyms also have childcare available.

Walking Program
Starting a regular walking program is a good choice because you can exercise anytime you choose, it does not cost anything and it can be adapted to your present physical condition. A walking program can be modified to meet your changing needs; it can be started, suspended, decreased or accelerated according to your physical energy.

Recommendations for a Walking Program:
- **Frequency:** Four times a week minimum, six times a week maximum; try not to skip more than one day in a row if your health allows.
- **Goal:** Gradually increase and maintain your heart rate at 100 – 120

Value of Exercise

beats per minute during your walk.
- **Duration:** Brisk walking at your own rate; start at 10 minutes per session and increase gradually to 30 minutes per session, as tolerated.
- **Location:** Preferably outdoors, when weather permits; indoor mall or treadmill.
- **Attire:** Comfortable shoes designed for walking and layered, loose, cotton clothing to absorb perspiration.
- **Equipment:** Consider purchasing a pedometer that measures the distance you walk and monitors your heart rate.
- **Evaluation:** Use the "talk test" to determine if the activity is too strenuous. During your exercise, you should be able to talk in sentences without feeling out of breath. If you cannot speak a full sentence, you should reduce your exercise level.
- **Precaution:** Stop any exercise if it causes or increases pain.

Walking Routine:
- Five minutes of slow walking to warm up.
- Increase walking at a brisk pace to increase heart rate to 100 – 120 beats per minute (take your pulse for 6 seconds and multiply by 10 to check your heart rate).
- Gradually increase the time your pulse remains at your target heart rate by extending your walk as tolerated. Walking should increase your energy after your heart rate returns to normal, without causing fatigue. Do not exercise to a point of exhaustion; this is not healthy and is not recommended.
- For the last five minutes, reduce your pace to allow your heart rate to gradually return to normal.

Walking Tips:
- Walk with a partner, if possible.
- Carry personal identification with you.
- Listen to your favorite music if you walk alone.
- Keep an exercise log or diary to monitor your progress.
- Exercise at the same time each day, if possible, to make walking a routine.
- Drink a full glass of water before and after you walk.
- Walk in a safe area, away from traffic.

Chapter 11

Exercise Evaluation

The ultimate test to evaluate whether you are overdoing your exercise is to wait one hour after completion and then ask yourself, *"Do I have more energy and feel more relaxed?"* If the answer is yes, you are exercising in a range that is building energy. If the answer is no, you are over-taxing your body's physical reserves, and you need to reduce the intensity or duration of your exercise.

Do Not Exercise if You Have:

- Fever
- Nausea or vomiting
- Muscle or joint pain with swelling
- Bleeding from any source
- Irregular heartbeat
- Dizziness or fainting
- Chest, arm or jaw pain
- Blood drawing on the same day (You may exercise afterward, but prior exercise may alter counts.)
- Any restrictions placed on exercise activities by a physician

Tips to Maintain Motivation

Exercise programs are often discontinued in a short time due to a lack of motivation. What keeps an individual motivated to continue an exercise program?

The first motivational factor is a strong change of belief in why you need to exercise. You have to keep foremost in your mind what exercise does for you. Write the benefits of exercise on a sticky note and list the changes you hope to experience. Place the benefits where you can see them every day as a reminder of why you are engaging in the activity.

Keep a written record of when and how long you exercise—how far you walked or the length of time you participated in an activity. A written record provides you with visual feedback. Another great way to receive feedback is with a wearable exercise monitoring device, such as a Fitbit®. This device tracks your steps and provides feedback about calories burned. There is also a free app, MyFitnessPal®, which allows you to keep a daily record of the food you eat and of your activity. If weight loss is a goal, this

Value of Exercise

is a great way to track food intake and monitor your calories. The site also has a blog offering helpful tips and support.

Recruit an exercise partner, join a team sport, join a gym, get a trainer or share a trainer with a friend. Accountability to someone else is a great motivator.

Reward yourself—a new pair of shoes after so many miles of walking, etc. You know what best motivates you.

Benefits of Exercise:
- Increased energy
- Increased physical endurance
- Increased capacity for healing
- Increased immunity
- Increased quality of sleep
- Decreased pain
- Decreased anxiety
- Decreased depression
- Increased sex drive
- Increase in weight control

The Value of Exercise

Fatigue is often addressed by getting additional rest. When in reality, too much rest promotes fatigue. Taking the opportunity to increase your energy through a regular program of exercise will pay high dividends in restoring your physical stamina and increasing your sex drive.

Chapter 11

Remember

- *Research confirms that too much physical rest can cause fatigue rather than relieving it.*
- *A balance between exercise and rest is essential for energy to be restored.*
- *Exercise promotes removal of the body's cellular waste. Muscular contractions around the lymphatic vessels move the waste into circulation for elimination from the body. Improved elimination of cellular waste increases overall health and decreases fatigue.*
- *Exercise increases your physical endurance, increases your capacity to heal, increases available energy, elevates mood, decreases pain, lowers anxiety, decreases depression and boosts immunity.*
- *Exercise, of your choice, is the key to regaining and increasing your energy and restoring your energy for sex.*

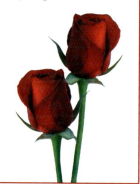

Chapter 12

Value of Nutrition

The season following cancer treatment is a perfect opportunity to slow down and reevaluate your life. Cancer serves as a wake-up call that allows a woman to evaluate what is important to her and serves as an opportunity to reorder priorities. At the top of the list of future desires is usually a goal to regain her health and have a strong, healthy body. Building a strong, healthy body for the future starts with the food you put into your body. In this chapter, we will discuss the basics of how to maximize your future health through diet.

As you recover, it is helpful to keep in mind that chemotherapy and radiation treatments killed cancerous cells and, in the process, also destroyed normal, healthy cells that need to be replaced. New cells are rebuilt from what you eat and drink. Rebuilding cells is a process that extends over a number of months. Therefore, for complete recovery to occur, it is important that you have the necessary nutrients to rebuild healthy cells.

The information in this chapter is not about restrictive diets, but about suggestions that are flexible and easy to incorporate into your normal lifestyle. I encourage you to consider your nutrition a vital part of your recovery. You alone can make these daily choices about what you eat. Deciding to eat nutritious foods is a gift only you can give yourself.

Weight Gain During Treatment

Some women who have had chemotherapy experience weight gain, and some do not. On average, women who undergo breast cancer treatment may experience weight gain of 10 – 15 pounds. Weight gain is most often caused by medications that change your hormonal balance or by medication given to block the estrogen in your body after treatment, such as tamoxifen or aromatase inhibitors (AIs). Inactivity during cancer treatment can also be a contributing factor. Some women respond to stress by eating more.

Chapter 12

Weight gain can contribute to lowered self-esteem and hinder sexual activity. If you find that you have gained weight, now is the time to begin making healthy choices. However, do not panic and go on a restrictive diet that could impact your continuing recovery. Don't allow the numbers on a scale to determine how you feel about yourself. Avoid weighing yourself daily. Sacrificing your health by extreme dieting to reach a certain number on the scale is not a smart health decision.

Eating for Future Health

Your goal after cancer treatment should be to rebuild your health by eating a nutritious, balanced diet, which maintains your body weight while not making you feel hungry or deprived. Now is not the time for fad diets, which often cut out specific food groups. You should not attempt any diet that causes extreme hunger or is highly restrictive. Restrictive diets do not promote recovery; they only increase stress, which is not good for you. The focus of this chapter is to provide guidelines and tips that will help you make better nutritional choices without the stress of a restrictive diet. Remember that with every food selection you make, you have the opportunity to give your body the fuel needed to rebuild healthy cells.

Nutrition Evaluation

The first step in smart eating is to evaluate your dietary habits to ensure that you are eating nutritious foods from all food groups and that you are not adding empty calories that could add to weight gain. The following tips offer simple changes that can easily be adapted to your lifestyle. The goal is to incorporate as many of the dietary tips as possible to maintain your energy and prevent unwanted weight gain.

Hunger Control Is Essential

When we get hungry, we tend to eat the first thing we find to satisfy that hunger. The first concept to understand is that it takes fewer calories to prevent hunger than it does to deal with it once it occurs. The goal is to prevent hunger.

Hunger Control Tips:
- Eat three, small balanced meals a day. Include nutritious snacks between meals to keep hunger at bay.
- Reducing portions and eating smaller meals throughout the day helps to curb hunger. Try eating five to six times a day. Going without food for

Value of Nutrition

several hours can lead to hypoglycemia (low blood sugar) which causes fatigue and slows your metabolism.

Stay Hydrated

When you feel as if you're starving, drink a large glass of cool water to help reduce the urge to snack. Drink lots of water throughout the day. Water (fluid intake) is crucial to your health. Water makes up about 60 percent of your body weight, and every system in your body depends on water to function properly. Lack of water can lead to dehydration, a condition that occurs when you don't have enough water in your body for your cells to carry on normal functions. Even mild dehydration can make you feel tired.

Early Signs and Symptoms of Dehydration:

- Thirst
- Fatigue
- Headache
- Dry mouth
- Muscle weakness
- Little or no urination
- Dizziness or lightheadedness

How Much Water Do You Need?

The average recommendation to maintain water balance is eight 8-ounce glasses per day. This amount should be increased when participating in activities that cause excessive sweating.

When You Don't Like Water

Some people do not like drinking plain water. The goal is to drink fluids that are not calorie dense and loaded with sugar. Sugary drinks quickly add weight and do not rebuild cells.

Tips for Making Water More Tasteful:

- Squeeze lemon into the water.
- Add whole strawberries or slices of cucumber, orange or lime to a pitcher of water and allow flavor to permeate.
- Add products like Emergen-C® (found in discount or health food stores). These products, which come in many flavors, can easily be added to a bottle of water to provide a healthy, energizing drink containing extra vitamin C, B vitamins and electrolytes, with very few calories.

Chapter 12

Eliminate Empty Liquid Calories:
- Avoid all sugary drinks when possible: soft drinks, sweetened tea, sweetened coffee drinks or sports drinks. These drinks are full of calories and cause a quick rise in blood sugar. They may provide a rush of energy, but the downside is that they cause blood sugar drops afterward, causing fatigue.
- Avoid diet drinks. They have been associated with weight gain in some people and add no nutritional value to your diet.
- Monitor the amount of fruit juice you drink because it is also high in calories. Choosing to eat the whole fruit is a better choice when possible. Eat an orange at breakfast rather than drinking a glass of orange juice.
- Select 100 percent vegetable or tomato juice, one percent or skim milk, soy milk, tea or coffee for lower-calorie choices.

Understanding Carbohydrates in Your Diet

Carbohydrates (carbs) are foods that when eaten and digested break down into glucose (sugar), which gives you energy. In the past few years, some of the diet fads have promoted low-carb diets for weight control. The goal following cancer treatment is to avoid fad diets and eat foods from all food groups, including carbohydrates. However, some carbohydrates are healthier choices than others for maintaining energy and weight control. They are identified through the glycemic index.

The glycemic index ranks carbohydrate foods by how much and how quickly they raise the blood sugar level, which is called the "glycemic response." Foods that raise glucose levels quickly have a higher glycemic index rating than foods that cause a slower rise. The lower the rating, the better the carbohydrate is to help control your appetite and lower your risk of diabetes. Lower-rated carbs are healthier choices because they are usually lower in calories and higher in fiber, nutrients and antioxidants.

Choosing low glycemic index foods may help you control your appetite because they tend to keep you feeling full longer. Other health benefits of low glycemic index foods include:

- Controls your blood glucose level by maintaining a more constant level of energy
- Controls your appetite by maintaining your blood sugar level
- Lowers your risk of getting heart disease by helping control your

Value of Nutrition

cholesterol level
- Lowers your risk of getting type 2 diabetes by keeping your blood sugar level lower

Glycemic Index Rating

Carbohydrates on the Glycemic Index Are Rated As:
- Low (55 or less)
- Medium (56 – 69)
- High (70 and over)

Your goal is to select lower glycemic foods. Selecting foods rated lower on the glycemic index helps you control hunger and blood sugar dips. This helps control weight.

Low Glycemic Foods (55 or Less):
- Skim milk
- Plain yogurt
- Soy beverage
- Apples/plums/oranges
- Sweet potato
- Oat bran bread
- Oatmeal (slow-cook oats)
- Bran cereal
- Converted or parboiled rice
- Pumpernickel bread
- Pasta
- Lentils (beans)
- Honey

Medium Glycemic Foods (56 – 69):
- Bananas, pineapples, raisins
- Popcorn
- Brown rice
- Shredded wheat cereal
- Whole wheat bread
- Rye bread

High Glycemic Foods (70 and over):
- Dried dates, watermelon
- Instant mashed potatoes
- Baked white potato
- Instant rice
- Corn Flakes®; Rice Krispies®; Cheerios®
- Bagel, white
- Soda crackers
- Jelly beans; candies
- French fries
- Ice cream
- Cookies
- Table sugar

Chapter 12

Maximize Good Carbohydrates

Good carbs are lower on the glycemic index and include beans and grains. Their fiber content will fill you up while promoting healthy blood sugar levels.

Beans

- Beans are also filled with nutrients and phytochemicals (plant chemicals) that have been shown to be active in the prevention of diseases.
- Beans are inexpensive, easy to prepare and last for several days when refrigerated. They can be eaten alone, with brown rice or added to soups, salads or stews. Aim for one-half cup serving or more of beans each day.
- The best bean choices include: soybeans, lentils, kidney beans, chickpeas (garbanzo), butter beans, navy beans, black beans, white beans or split peas.

Grains

- Do not deprive yourself of bread and cereal; just make sure that you choose 100 percent whole grains—whole wheat, whole oats, brown rice, rye, barley, etc.
- When buying grain products look for the phrase "whole grain."

Vegetables and Fruits

- Vegetables are low in calories and high in fiber. Vegetables are natural appetite suppressants because they are very filling and are packed with vitamins, minerals and phytochemicals.
- The best vegetable choices include: cabbage, kale, broccoli, cauliflower, Brussels sprouts, collards, carrots, garlic, onions, leeks, tomatoes, asparagus, spinach, dark varieties of lettuce, red or orange bell peppers.
- Try to limit or avoid the high glycemic index or starchy vegetables such as corn, white potatoes, parsnips and rutabagas, which raise your blood sugar quickly.
- Fruits are highly nutritious. Strive to include two servings a day.
- If you are watching your weight, the best fruit options include berries (any variety), cherries, plums, any whole citrus, cantaloupe, grapes, peaches, apples, pears, dried or fresh apricots.
- Limit the amount of higher glycemic fruits such as bananas, mangoes, papaya, pineapple, raisins and dates.

VALUE OF NUTRITION

Healthy Proteins:
- Proteins provide a steady, prolonged blood glucose level with minimal insulin response and will keep you feeling satisfied longer between meals.
- Healthy proteins include fish (oily varieties such as salmon, tuna, mackerel, sardines, herring and trout), shellfish, skinless poultry, nuts, seeds, soy, wild game, lean dairy products (cottage cheese and yogurt), beans/legumes and eggs.
- Limit other protein sources such as red meat or pork to two servings a week.
- Eating protein at breakfast is especially important for energy and weight control.

Fats
- Newer dietary studies have shown the important role of dietary fat. The body requires adequate fat to repair cells. It is important to eat good sources of dietary fat.
- Dietary fat makes food taste better, satisfies your appetite and reduces hunger.
- Many of the good fats are found in the sources of protein listed above. Additional sources include extra virgin olive oil, canola oil, nuts, seeds, coconut oil and avocados.
- Avoid trans fats. These are vegetable oils that have been processed, such as margarine and shortening.
- Minimize saturated fats found in fatty cuts of beef, pork or lamb.
- Green salads with olive oil dressing are an excellent way to get a healthy serving of fat.

Nuts:
- Unsalted, unprocessed nuts are a great source of protein. They make an easy, healthy snack because they contain protein and are nutritionally dense.
- Walnuts, almonds, cashews, pistachios, hazelnuts, Brazil nuts, pecans and pine nuts are good choices.
- Include 1 – 1.5 ounces of nuts in your daily diet. Buy raw nuts in bulk and divide into smaller packages to carry as a handy snack.

Chapter 12

Portion Sizes To Control Weight

When eating a meal, limit portion sizes at any one sitting to no more than the equivalent of your hands cupped together. The exception to this rule is non-starchy vegetables, which can be eaten in large amounts.

Healthy Eating Preparation

Eating right requires being prepared. When you are hungry, or when your energy is low, it is easy to eat the most convenient food rather than making a healthy choice.

- Purchase and have healthy foods, snacks and drinks available.
- Stock your pantry and freezer with an assortment of healthy foods.
- Cook several meals and freeze them for the days when you don't feel up to cooking.
- Buy large packages of nuts and whole grain crackers and divide them into small plastic bags.
- Keep small amounts of food in your stomach to help prevent hunger and fatigue caused by low blood sugar.
- Carry water and a healthy snack of nuts, fruit or whole wheat crackers with you to avoid getting hungry when away from home. Don't get caught without something nutritious to eat.

Nutrition After Cancer Treatment Tips:
- Make every spoonful and every drink you take count nutritionally. Your body is building healthy new cells to replace those damaged by chemotherapy.
- Eat five to six small meals rather than three large ones. Small meals are better tolerated.
- Because your body is building new cells, it is essential to get adequate protein. Good protein choices include whole wheat bread or crackers combined with peanut butter, almond butter (tastes like peanut butter and is highly nutritious), hard-boiled eggs, yogurt, liquid yogurt or cottage cheese.
- Limit the amount of fluid you drink during meals to avoid getting full too quickly. Drink between meals instead. Adequate fluid intake and staying hydrated are essential. Monitor your intake to be sure you are getting enough fluids. Filling a bottle with your daily intake of water

Value of Nutrition

at the beginning of the day will help you monitor how much you are drinking.
- Make high-protein smoothies in a blender out of yogurt, fresh fruit or peanut or almond butter. Smoothies are a smart way to get lots of protein while avoiding the hassle of food preparation.

Building Energy Through Nutrition

What you eat and how you move your body are predictors of how much energy you will have in the future. Eating nutritious food and getting regular exercise are keys to increasing your energy and improving your mood. When your body has nutrients available and the ability to transport oxygen to all of its cells, this increases the body's capacity to heal, increases available energy, elevates mood, decreases pain, lowers anxiety, decreases depression and boosts immunity. The extra bonus is that when your energy increases, so will your sex life.

Plan to make changes in your diet that will enhance your recovery. These are changes that no one can make for you. Making good food choices is a habit. The good news is that bad habits can be broken, and new habits can be developed. If you recognize that there are changes that may benefit you, now is the time to plan what you need to change and when to get started. If you find change hard to stick with, enlist a friend or support partner to join you or be your cheerleader. You will never regret these positive changes. These changes are a gift that you can give yourself.

CHAPTER 12

Remember

- *Do not select a diet to lose weight; instead, select a diet to create health.*

- *Diets that limit the amount of food eaten and create hunger are psychologically stressful and should always be avoided.*

- *Do not allow the numbers on a bathroom scale to dictate how you feel about yourself.*

- *Concentrate on choosing foods that will give your body the nutrients needed to rebuild healthy cells.*

- *An energetic, healthy body is the foundation of an active, robust sex life.*

Chapter 13

The Single Woman and Future Sexual Intimacy

Following cancer treatment, sexuality issues present a unique challenge for the single, divorced or widowed woman. Not only do they have to deal with body image changes and lingering treatment side effects, but they also have to deal with the psychological issues of developing future intimacy with a new partner. After cancer treatment, some women in our focus groups reported they felt as if they were damaged goods and would not be sexually attractive as a partner. This is not true! Many single women have successfully developed intimate relationships after cancer treatment.

If you are single and are having these negative thoughts, I want you to rethink these thoughts. A cancer diagnosis does not define who you are. You are still the same person—you just happened to have an experience with cancer. After undergoing cancer treatment, most patients emerge much stronger and more sensitive. The cancer experience, instead of diminishing your value, served to make you a more attractive person. The cancer experience increases your maturity in relationships, which enables you to become a better person, friend and lover. As we have discussed throughout this book, a good sex life comes from a good relationship.

The first necessary step is to make peace with yourself about your diagnosis. Cancer is a life event that no one would ever seek to experience in their life, but it is an event that quickly allows an individual to learn what is really important in life. The diagnosis serves as a catalyst to redefine important and non-important life events. Often, things that seemed essential or desired before the diagnosis move into the non-important category after diagnosis.

Chapter 13

One woman shared, *"Cancer helped me to no longer focus on issues that were minor but instead to focus on those that were of value. A bad hair day when compared to a day of no hair from chemo, no longer shook my world. I now had a comparison as to what was really important."* Maturity about life is a positive by-product of having lived through a cancer diagnosis.

Remember, to a new partner you offer a unique value of maturity that is often not present in people who have not had their life tested by adversity. Your value has not diminished; it has increased!

Future Dating Considerations:
- The largest roadblock when reentering the dating world is what YOU think about yourself. You are not damaged goods. You are a person with increased value because of successfully mastering the crisis of a cancer diagnosis.
- You are not alone. One-third of all Americans will have a cancer diagnosis in their lifetime. Approximately one-half of those diagnosed will be single, divorced or widowed.
- Dating after cancer treatment will be the same as it was before treatment. Dating was not always successful before cancer, and it will not always be successful after cancer. If a new relationship does not work out, don't blame you cancer experience or receive it as a personal rejection. When a relationship does not progress, it usually has nothing to do with your cancer history; instead, it is simply the nature of new relationships and dating.

Sharing Your Cancer Experience

One of the biggest challenges single women face is when and how they will tell a new partner about their cancer experience. Understanding how other women have handled this issue will give you a sense of direction on how to prepare and will allow you to develop your own plan for sharing. Surround yourself with understanding peers as you work through the process of preparing what you will say in the future.

The best time to share is when the relationship has passed the mutual friendship stage and is beginning to progress. However, you should share this information before the relationship becomes serious, or if you think that intimacy may occur. Only you will know when it is the right time.

THE SINGLE WOMAN AND FUTURE SEXUAL INTIMACY

Tips for Sharing Your Experience:
- When you feel the time is right, select a time and place where you will feel comfortable discussing your cancer history. Select a place where you will not feel embarrassed if you become upset.
- Begin the conversation by explaining that you desire respect and honesty in your relationships and that you have something important you need to share.
- Explain the facts about your diagnosis honestly and openly:
  - *"In (year) I was diagnosed with (type of cancer).*
  - *My diagnosis required that I have a (mastectomy, lumpectomy, etc.) that was followed by (type of treatments).*
  - *I have been cancer free for (time).*
    or
    I am currently dealing with (problems).
  - *I feel that what I went through has allowed me to become a stronger person because I have had to deal with a lot of hard issues.*
  - *I wanted to be very honest with you before this relationship progresses. I will be happy to answer any questions you have about my diagnosis, treatment or present health."*
- Do not appear as a victim; you want their care and concern, not their pity.
- Ask the other person what they think about what you just told them.
- Allow the other person time to talk about their feelings and to ask questions.

Remember, if this person leaves the relationship after you share details about your cancer experience, this is a person who likely would have deserted you in the future during hard times. You did yourself a favor by sharing early in the relationship. You have likely prevented future heartache. Some relationships work, and some don't. Your goal is to emotionally protect yourself by sharing early enough to find out if this information will impact the relationship before you fall in love.

As a single woman, you need to be prepared to deal with discussing your diagnosis with future partners with confidence. Cancer has not damaged you; it has been a tool for expanding your ability to love and appreciate life. You deserve a partner who has the same level of personal maturity.

Chapter 13

Remember

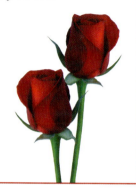

- *Being diagnosed with cancer does not change who you are.*
- *A cancer diagnosis can serve to make a person stronger and more sensitive.*
- *You are not damaged goods.*
- *You are a person who has an expanded ability to love and appreciate life.*
- *Your value has not diminished because of cancer; it has increased!*

Chapter 14

Drugs That Lower Your Sex Drive

One of the reasons for low sex drive may be the medication(s) you are taking. Prescription medications are one of the top causes of sex drive reduction. If you are attempting to increase your sex drive, it is essential to know which medications the manufacturers indicate may have reduced desire as a side effect.

Sex Drive-Reducing Medication Categories:
- Hormonal contraceptions (birth control pills, patches or a Mirena IUD)
- Hormone-blocking medications (tamoxifen, aromatase inhibitors)
- Synthetic hormone replacement medications
- Psychiatric medications (prescribed for depression, anxiety, bipolar disorder, obsessive-compulsive disorder, ADHD, schizophrenia)
- Anti-seizure medications
- Blood pressure medications
- Cholesterol-lowering medications
- Sleep medications
- Pain medications

To help you determine whether you are taking a medication that has the potential to reduce your sex drive, we have included the names of medications whose manufacturers have indicated reduced libido (sex drive) as a possible side effect on page 118. If you are taking medication, look for the name of your medication on the list to see if sex drive reduction may be a potential side effect. This list is from the *PDR* (*Physicians' Desk Reference*), a medication side-effect reference guide used by physicians.

Chapter 14

If you are taking a medication on the list, it may be possible to change to another medication in the same drug class, which can have a different effect on your sex drive. Ask your physician about trying another medication. Simply switching from one medication to another in the same class may solve the problem of reduced sex drive.

Impact of Recreational Drugs on Sexuality

Recreational drugs can also have an impact on sexual desire. Marijuana reduces inhibitions and alters consciousness, causing the perception of increased sexual performance; however, regular use lowers testosterone levels, which negatively impacts future levels of desire.

Impact of Alcohol on Sexuality

Beverages containing alcohol may make you feel amorous when it comes to sex, but too much alcohol can reduce your sex drive. When under the influence of alcohol, an individual feels more sexual and has a stronger desire to seek out a sexual experience only to find that alcohol inhibits sexual performance. In low doses, alcohol helps alleviate the anxiety about sexual performance and sexuality. However, when alcohol is chronically consumed over a long period, it limits a person's sexual function and performance.

Tamoxifen and Aromatase Inhibitor Medication Therapy

Tamoxifen or an aromatase inhibitor is routinely prescribed as part of post-treatment therapy for estrogen receptor-positive breast cancer patients to reduce the risk of cancer recurrence. In the past, patients were placed on endocrine therapy (tamoxifen or an aromatase inhibitor) for five years to reduce their risk of cancer recurrence. New recommendations have changed to extend the length of time from five to ten years. Tamoxifen and aromatase inhibitors both have sexual side effects, with aromatase inhibitors having the greatest impact on sexual dysfunction. Continuing to deal with the sexual side effects of these medications for an additional five years proves challenging for some patients. The good news is that there is a new study, The Breast Cancer Index (BCI), that can help a woman determine whether or not she will likely benefit from extending hormonal therapy for an additional five years.

Drugs That Lower Your Sex Drive

New Test to Predict Benefit of Extended Endocrine Therapy
The Breast Cancer Index^{SM} study is designed for estrogen receptor-positive/lymph node negative patients who have taken endocrine therapy (tamoxifen or aromatase inhibitor) for four to five years. The study helps determine the benefit a patient may have by continuing to take an endocrine therapy for an additional five years.

The BCI study is performed using the original tumor pathology slides to analyze the tumor gene expression; from this expression, it predicts the risk of late cancer recurrence. The BCI test reports the future risk of cancer recurrence on a scale of low risk, intermediate risk or high risk. This predictive projection allows you and your physician to evaluate the likelihood of receiving benefit from continuing endocrine therapy for an additional five years. Women whose recurrence score results are low are unlikely to benefit from extended endocrine therapy. This information may allow you to confidently stop taking endocrine therapy after five years and avoid the unwanted side effects of continuing the medication.

If you have been on endocrine therapy and are approaching your fifth year, you qualify to have the study performed on your pathology slides. Ask your doctor about the BCI study to evaluate your status. The BCI study results will aid you and your physician in making an individualized decision about future care. The decision to continue or not to continue taking endocrine therapy should be made in correlation with other clinical findings.

Additional information about the Breast Cancer Index study is available at www.breastcancerindex.com.

Chapter 14

Possible Medication Side Effect: Decreased Libido

- Abilify Tablets (Infrequent)
- Aciphex Tablets
- Actiq (Less than 1%)
- Adalat CC Tablets (Less than 1%)
- Adderall XR Capsules (2% to 4%)
- Aldoclor Tablets
- Aldoril Tablets
- Ambien Tablets (Rare)
- Amerge Tablets (Rare)
- Anadrol-50 Tablets
- AndroGel (Up to 3%)
- Antara Capsules
- Aricept Tablets (Infrequent)
- Aricept ODT Tablets (Infrequent)
- Asacol Delayed-Release Tablets
- Avinza Capsules (Less than 5%)
- Avodart Soft Gelatin Capsules (0.3% to 3%)
- Axid Oral Solution
- Blocadren Tablets (0.6%)
- Caduet Tablets (Less than 2%)
- Calcijex Injection
- Campral Tablets (Frequent)
- Casodex Tablets (2% to 5%)
- Celexa (2%)
- Clozapine Tablets (Less than 1%)
- Clozaril Tablets (Less than 1%)
- Copaxone for Injection (Infrequent)
- Coreg Tablets (Greater than 0.1% to 1%)
- Cosopt Sterile Ophthalmic Solution
- Cozaar Tablets (Less than 1%)
- Cymbalta Delayed-Release Capsules (1% to 6%)
- Delatestryl Injection
- Depo-Provera Contraceptive Injection (1% to 5%)
- Depo-SubQ Provera 104 Injectable Suspension (1% to less than 5%)
- Diovan HCT Tablets (Greater than 0.2%)
- Duragesic Transdermal System (Less than 1%)
- DynaCirc CR Tablets (0.5% to 1%)
- Effexor Tablets (2% to 5.7%)
- Effexor XR Capsules (3% to 9%)
- Eligard 7.5 mg (Less than 2%)
- Eligard 30 mg (3.3%)
- Eligard 45 mg (1%)
- Exelon Capsules (Infrequent)
- FazaClo Orally Disintegrating Tablets (Less than 1%)
- Flomax Capsules (1.0% to 2.0%)
- Gabitril Tablets (Infrequent)
- Gengraf Capsules (1% to less than 3%)
- Hectorol Capsules
- Hectorol Injection
- Hyperstat I.V. Injection
- Hytrin Capsules (0.6%)
- Hyzaar
- Imdur Tablets (Less than or equal to 5%)
- Indapamide Tablets (Less than 5%)
- Infergen (5%)
- Intron A for Injection (Up to 5%)
- Inversine Tablets
- Kadian Capsules (Less than 3%)
- Kaletra (Up to 2%)
- Klonopin (1%)
- Lamictal (Rare)
- Lexapro Oral Solution (3% to 7%)
- Lexapro Tablets (3% to 7%)

Drugs That Lower Your Sex Drive

- Librium Capsules
- Lipitor Tablets (Less than 2%)
- Lofibra Capsules
- Lotensin HCT Tablets (0.3% to 1%)
- Lotrel Capsules
- Lunesta Tablets (0% to 3%)
- Lupron Depot 3.75 mg (Less than 5%)
- Lupron Depot 7.5 mg (5.4%)
- Lupron Depot-3 Month 11.25 mg (1.8% to 11%)
- Lyrica Capsules (Greater than or equal to 1%)
- Mavik Tablets (0.3% to 1.0%)
- Megace ES Oral Suspension (0% to 5%)
- Meridia Capsules
- Midamor Tablets (Less than or equal to 1%)
- Mirapex Tablets (1%)
- Mirena Intrauterine System (5% or more)
- Moduretic Tablets
- MS Contin Tablets (Less frequent)
- Nadolol Tablets (1 to 5 of 1000 patients)
- Neoral Soft Gelatin Capsules (1% to less than 3%)
- Neoral Oral Solution (1% to less than 3%)
- Neurontin Capsules (Infrequent)
- Neurontin Oral Solution (Infrequent)
- Neurontin Tablets (Infrequent)
- Niravam Orally Disintegrating Tablets (14.4%)
- Norvir (Less than 2%)
- OxyContin Tablets
- Pacerone Tablets (1% to 3%)
- Paxil CR Controlled-Release Tablets (3% to 9%)
- Paxil (3% to 9%)
- Pepcid Injection (Infrequent)
- Pepcid (Infrequent)
- Permax Tablets (Infrequent)
- Plendil Extended-Release Tablets (0.5% to 1.5%)
- Prevacid Delayed-Release Capsules (Less than 1%)
- Prevacid for Delayed-Release Oral Suspension (Less than 1%)
- Prevacid NapraPAC (Less than 1%)
- Prevacid SoluTab Delayed-Release Orally Disintegrating Tablets (Less than 1%)
- PREVPAC (Less than 1%)
- Prinivil Tablets (0.4%)
- Prinzide Tablets (0.3% to 1%)
- Prochieve 4% Gel (10%)
- Prochieve 8% Gel (10%)
- Propecia Tablets (1.8% - 6.4%)
- Proscar Tablets (2.6% to 6.4%)
- ProSom Tablets (Rare)
- Protonix I.V. (Less than 1%)
- Protonix Tablets (Less than 1%)
- Provigil Tablets (At least 1%)
- Prozac Pulvules and Liquid (1% to 11%)
- Requip Tablets (Infrequent)
- Rescriptor Tablets
- Reyataz Capsules (Less than 3%)
- Rilutek Tablets (Infrequent)
- Risperdal Consta Long-Acting Injection (Infrequent)
- Rythmol SR Capsules
- Sandostatin Injection (Less than 1%)
- Sandostatin LAR Depot (Rare)
- Seroquel Tablets (Rare)
- Sonata Capsules (Infrequent)
- Soriatane Capsules (Less than 1%)
- Strattera Capsules (5% or greater)
- Sular Tablets (Less than or equal to 1%)

Chapter 14

- Surmontil Capsules
- Symbyax Capsules (2% to 4%)
- Symmetrel (0.1% to 1%)
- Tambocor Tablets (Less than 1%)
- Tarka Tablets
- Tasmar Tablets (Infrequent)
- Thalomid Capsules
- Timolide Tablets (Less than 1%)
- Timoptic in Ocudose
- Timoptic Sterile Ophthalmic Solution
- Timoptic-XE Sterile Ophthalmic Gel Forming-Solution
- Topamax Sprinkle Capsules (0% to 3%)
- Topamax Tablets (0% to 3%)
- Toprol-XL Tablets
- Trelstar LA Suspension (2.3%)
- Tricor Tablets
- Trileptal Oral Suspension
- Trileptal Tablets
- Uniretic Tablets (Less than 1%)
- Vantas (2.3%)
- Vaseretic Tablets (0.5% to 2.0%)
- VFEND I.V. (Less than 2%)
- VFEND Oral Suspension (Less than 2%)
- VFEND Tablets (Less than 2%)
- Vicoprofen Tablets (Less than 1%)
- Wellbutrin Tablets (3.1%)
- Wellbutrin SR Sustained-Release Tablets (Infrequent)
- Wellbutrin XL Extended-Release Tablets (Infrequent)
- Xanax XR Tablets (6%)
- Zantac Injection
- Zantac Injection Pharmacy Bulk Packaging (Infrequent)
- Zestoretic Tablets (0.3% to 1%)
- Zestril Tablets (0.4%)
- Zoladex (61%)
- Zoloft (1% to 11%)
- Zonegran Capsules (Infrequent)
- Zyban Sustained-Release Tablets (Infrequent)
- Zyprexa Tablets (Infrequent)
- Zyprexa ZYDIS Orally Disintegrating Tablets (Infrequent)
- Zyrtec Chewable Tablets (Less than 2%)
- Zyrtec (Less than 2%)
- Zyrtec-D 12 Hour Extended Release Tablets (Less than 2%)

Possible Medication Side Effect: Loss of Libido

- Advicor Tablets
- Altoprev Extended-Release Tablets
- Catapres Tablets (About 3 in 100 patients)
- Catapres-TTS (0.5% or less)
- Clorpres Tablets (About 3%)
- Eulexin Capsules (36%)
- Klonopin (Infrequent)
- Lescol Capsules
- Lescol XL Tablets
- Mevacor Tablets (0.5% to 1.0%)
- Orap Tablets
- Pravachol Tablets
- Roferon-A Injection (Infrequent)
- Vytorin 10/10 Tablets
- Vytorin 10/20 Tablets
- Vytorin 10/40 Tablets
- Vytorin 10/80 Tablets
- Zantac (Occasional)
- Zocor Tablets

DRUGS THAT LOWER YOUR SEX DRIVE

Remember

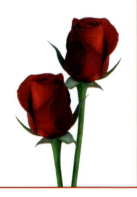

- *You may experience reduced sex drive due to medication.*
- *Check to see if the medication(s) you are taking is on the list of drugs in this chapter. These are drugs that the manufacturers indicate may reduce sexual desire.*
- *If your medication is listed, talk to your doctor about changing your medication to one which does not impact sexual desire.*
- *Alcohol can increase desire, but reduces sexual arousal and the ability to experience an orgasm.*

Chapter 15

Understanding Female Sex Drive

One of the most frequently misunderstood issues regarding female sexuality is the female sex drive and sexual response. What women most often know about female sex drive comes from what they have seen in movies and television shows or have read in books and magazines. In these media sources, the female is most often portrayed as a hottie who is eagerly seeking her next sexual encounter. When she finds a suitable partner, the media portrays her as becoming instantly aroused as she tears off her clothes and then passionately engages in mutually fulfilling sexual intercourse. Orgasm comes quickly and brings screams of delight and loud moaning, all occurring within a few minutes.

Regretfully, this media image of female sexuality has a strong influence on our idea of what our sex drive, sexual encounters, sexual arousal and sexual satisfaction should be like. When a woman's own personal experience does not equate the media portrayal, she may feel inadequate as a sexual partner. Her own sexual reality becomes clouded with doubt about her performance. What the media presents is a **false reality**. The media's portrayal of female sexuality is similar to their portrayal of "Barbie" being the **ideal** body type—with her thin body, long legs and large breasts. Neither the media's portrayal of sexual performance or the ideal body type of Barbie is realistic.

Often, our sexual partners have also been tutored by the same media portrayal of a sexual encounter. They, too, believe this is the model to follow. This leads to unrealistic expectations about response and performance. This mistruth causes sexual relationships to become a challenge and end in an unsatisfying sexual encounter—frustrating both partners.

Chapter 15

The portrayal of sexuality in the media has presented a false concept of female sexuality that greatly impacts many sexual relationships. This leads to the question, *"What is normal female sexual arousal and sexual satisfaction?"*

Normal Female Sex Drive

The reality is that the average female is not actively seeking a sexual encounter. The sex drive of the female is unlike the sex drive of the male. For most men, the sex drive is high and is driven by frequent sexual thoughts. These thoughts cause a male to be a consistent seeker of sexual encounters. Male sex drive is fueled by high levels of the hormone testosterone. In comparison, the average female's sex drive is not driven by high hormonal levels of testosterone promoting frequent sexual thoughts and quick sexual arousal.

Female Arousal Medication Challenge

One of the questions often asked about low female sexual desire is, *"Why isn't there a female Viagra®?"* That is a good question. The answer is that a woman's sexuality is more complex than male sexuality. Viagra® only addresses blood flow. For males, increased blood flow promotes an erection. An erection serves as sexual stimulation for a male. For women, increased blood flow is simply not enough. The **mind** of a woman must also be positively engaged.

In a female, brain chemistry is the major determining factor to full sexual arousal. A woman can be physically aroused with adequate blood flow to the genitals, but still not be interested in a sexual encounter depending on her brain's perception of the encounter and brain chemistry. A Viagra®-like drug that enhances only physical arousal through blood flow will not help because it does not address the complex issues of the mind.

Over the years, drug companies have spent hundreds of millions of dollars to find a female arousal drug. They've created drugs for women that function in the same basic fashion as male erection enhancers. These medications physically stimulated genitalia with increased blood flow but did not address the brain chemistry of sexual desire. Attempting to increase female sexual desire with a medication that only increases blood flow has been unsuccessful.

Understanding Female Sex Drive

Because of the psychological and physical connection, sex drive is more complicated for women than for men. Factors other than just physical functioning combine to create a woman's sex drive. Even the reason for participating in sexual activity differs in males and females. While males may want to be emotionally close to their partner, the main sexual drive is physical. A female's reasons for participating in sexual activity include the desire to be emotionally close to a partner, to show love and affection, to increase her sense of attractiveness to her mate, to share physical pleasure simply for the sake of sharing, and, only occasionally, is it to satisfy her own hormonally-driven sexual urge.

New Female Sexual Desire-Enhancing Medication

Recently the FDA approved the first non-hormonal, desire-enhancing drug for women. This medication, Addyi® (flibanserin), alters brain chemistry as the mechanism to increase desire rather than increasing blood flow. However, at present, the drug is minimally effective. Additional information on Addyi® is located in *Chapter 17: Desire-Enhancing Medications and Supplements.*

Role of the Brain in Sexual Desire

Before female sexual arousal occurs, sexual stimulation by a partner (touch, words) is first processed by the brain to determine whether the initiated sexual activity is an acceptable and desirable activity to pursue. Several factors can block or greatly impact a female's sexual desire during this processing.

The current relationship with the sexual partner is a major determining factor for sexual desire to progress to the next stage. Females, unlike males, have difficulty participating in fulfilling sex if their relationship with their partner is strained. Sex for a female is very dependent upon a healthy relationship. For this reason, the first "fix" for a good sexual relationship is to develop a good relational bond with your mate. If a relationship has a history of repeated stressful relational encounters, this often requires the help of an outside counselor. A counselor can help a couple work through their past and current relationship problems.

The second factor is past sexual encounters that have created a negative or painful experience. Past painful or negative sexual experiences can have a negative influence on the desire to participate in sexual activity. Women

Chapter 15

who have a history of sexual violation through molestation or rape may have trouble in their present sexual relationship. If you have a difficult sexual history and are struggling, counseling has proven very successful in identifying and removing these negative roadblocks.

If painful sex was experienced in the past, it puts a damper on future desire. It is necessary to address and correct vaginal dryness so sex will not be painful. Liberal use of lubricants, even after vaginal dryness is treated, is essential during intercourse to ensure adequate lubrication. If sex has been painful in the past, discuss your plan to restore the health of your vagina with your partner as outlined in *Chapter 5: Vaginal Dryness and Painful Intercourse*. It is necessary that sex not cause pain for future sexual desire to be spontaneous.

The third factor is present fears. Addressing fears of unwanted pregnancy or sexually transmitted disease is also essential. If pregnancy is a possibility, discuss the most appropriate method of birth control with your physician. In an established relationship, sexually transmitted disease issues have usually been resolved; but, in a new relationship, you should address this issue with your partner and take necessary steps to protect your health.

Female desire is dependent upon overcoming any psychological concerns for sexual activity to be pleasurable. The brain plays a huge role in determining whether sexual stimulation from a partner is an acceptable activity. After processing, the brain provides either a "green light" for arousal to proceed or a "red light" for the arousal process to stop. If you identify any psychological blocks that may impede your sexual desire, begin to take steps to correct them.

Female Sex Drive Enhancement

Physically, the female sex drive can be stimulated through appropriate, affectionate touch. Mentally, the female sex drive can be stimulated by words spoken to her or by memories of sights, smells or music that are personally associated with previous pleasant sexual experiences. Once mental and physical pathways are stimulated, the female sex drive builds slowly. Increased interest allows heightened sexual arousal to occur. Let's examine the process of female sexual arousal step-by-step.

Understanding Female Sex Drive

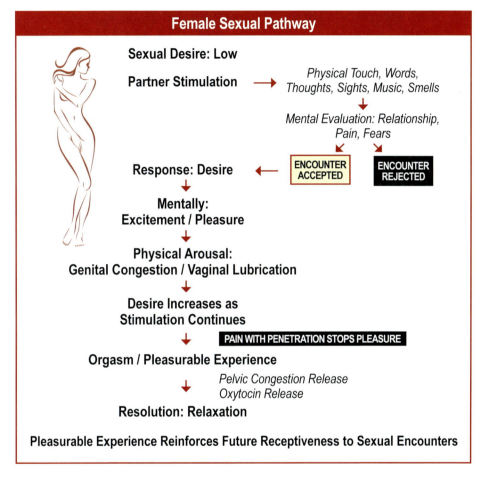

- Sexual stimulation is first processed by the female brain to validate that the stimulus (words, thoughts or physical touch) is acceptable and desired. The thoughts, *"Is it safe to proceed?"* or *"Do I want to proceed?"* are mentally processed. If the answer is yes, the brain clears the pathways to allow further sexual stimulation to proceed. Changes occur throughout the body—the genitals, muscles surrounding the vaginal canal, breasts, blood pressure and breath rate. The full body becomes engaged. If the answer to the sexual advance is no, a woman finds it difficult to continue and mentally and physically disengages in the process.
- With further loving, affirming words or physical touch, sexual arousal increases gradually. The blood flow increases to all the genital tissues,

Chapter 15

causing engorgement of the genitals (congestion). Congestion occurs when the smooth muscle cells around the blood spaces in the vulva, clitoris and vagina dilate, which allows the blood flow to increase and remain in the tissues, causing enlargement. The breasts also become congested with blood and enlarge and the nipples become erect. After the blood flow increases and causes congestion, a woman feels a pleasant tingling or throbbing in the genitals and the breasts become more sensitive to touch, which increases sexual pleasure.
- During this time of sexual foreplay, the vaginal wall secretes a slippery fluid that lubricates the vagina causing a woman to feel wet.
- The state of genital congestion and lubrication signals readiness for the sexual encounter. For vaginal intercourse to be comfortable and pleasurable, the female vagina must be adequately lubricated. Cancer-treated or menopausal women have difficulty lubricating sufficiently and require a sexual lubricant to prevent penetrative intercourse from being painful. If any discomfort occurs, stop immediately and apply additional lubricant.
- Orgasm may occur when peak excitement is reached. Orgasm consists of contractions of the pelvic muscles, which occur at approximately 0.8 second intervals. These contractions are followed by a slow release of the congestion in the pelvic area.
- Orgasm causes the release of the hormones prolactin and oxytocin. Prolactin is a hormone best known for promoting milk production. Oxytocin is a hormone best known as the bonding hormone, which causes feelings of closeness. These hormones combine after heightened sexual excitement to cause feelings of well-being, relaxation and a fatigue feeling after orgasm called resolution.

It is important to know that participating in sexual activity, even without orgasm promotes the same release and increase of the hormones oxytocin and prolactin. This hormonal upsurge increases feelings of satisfaction, closeness and pleasure.

What does this information mean to you when restoring your sex drive and creating a satisfying sexual relationship? It means that you must purposefully plan to increase your mental readiness for openness to sexual encounters. Address any issues in the relationship with your partner, treat vaginal dryness, address issues of unwanted pregnancy and your need for

Understanding Female Sex Drive

privacy. Addressing these issues helps remove the psychological barriers that can reduce desire.

You need to learn how to prime your sexual pump by learning what creates sexual excitement for you. Since most females are not aroused spontaneously, we must learn to create our own sexual stimuli. We should learn how to flip our sexual switch by understanding what turns us on. We have to share these things with our partner. We must schedule sex and make sexual encounters a priority. Scheduling sex probably does not sound very sexy, but when we put a date night on our schedule, it helps us plan and prepare our mind and body.

Women with older male partners need to remember that their partner may also need a scheduled date night so that they, too, can plan to be ready. Older partners who are also dealing with lower levels of sex hormones may also need time to prepare for sex. The partner may require preparation for sexual intimacy by taking Cialas® or Viagra®.

Sexual Mood Enhancement

Sounds:
- Prepare a list of your favorite love songs. Purchase CDs or download the music onto your iPod or phone so you can have easy access to them in the bathroom or bedroom. Hearing your favorite love songs can prompt the brain and be a signal to prepare for a sexual encounter.

Smells:
- Purchase essential oils or scented candles. Fill your room with pleasant smells that you find sexually stimulating (ylang ylang, lavender, sandalwood, etc.).
- Purchase bath oil, perfume or scented lotion for yourself.
- Purchase cologne or scented soaps that you find stimulating for your partner.

Touch:
- Purchase silky lingerie or a soft, luxurious bathrobe that you can slip into after your bath.
- Purchase high-quality soft or silky sheets for your bed.
- Purchase massage oil.

Chapter 15

- Purchase a vaginal lubricant.
- Take a warm bath with bath oil while burning scented candles and listening to your selected love songs.

Lighting:
- Determine what type of lighting you prefer in the bedroom—a lamp with a low-voltage bulb or candles.

Partner Communication

Now that you have prepared by purchasing items to enhance your sexual experience, let your partner know what turns on your sexual senses. Your partner needs to know what you find stimulating. Don't make this a guessing game. Your partner will appreciate knowing your sexual preferences.

I Am Most Turned On By:
- Being touched and caressed gently.
- Receiving a sensual massage from my partner.
- Smelling cologne or essential oils on their body after a shower.
- Hearing sweet words whispered into my ear.
- Listening to love music.
- Watching a sexy movie together.

Remove Environmental Distractions

On your scheduled date night, be sure you have a safe, quiet place where you will not be distracted. Women are very easily distracted by their external environment. Plan to have as much privacy as possible. Plan for small children to spend the night with a friend or family member if possible. Line up activities outside the home for teenage children. Put a lock on your bedroom door.

Tips to Increase Oxytocin

As we discussed, oxytocin is a feel good hormone. When oxytocin is released, it reduces stress and creates a calming effect. Increasing the level of oxytocin influences a person's mood. It generates more positive feelings toward others, which results in feelings of closeness and connectivity. Fear is also reduced. Increasing oxytocin is an effective way to protect oneself from, as well as to help treat, existing depression or anxiety.

Understanding Female Sex Drive

Oxytocin, produced by both females and males, has a number of health-promoting benefits. It has been shown to promote an increase in immunity and promote faster wound healing. Studies have also shown that oxytocin helps to reduce pain and lower blood pressure.

How can you increase your oxytocin level? Oxytocin levels rise after sexual intercourse. The great news is that oxytocin release can also be stimulated with other activities, which include loving and touching activities.

Remember the loving, close feelings of exhilaration you shared when you first met and developed a relationship with your partner? Somehow, over time, long-term relationships often lose their spontaneity in showing acts of love, including loving touch. Reduced showing-of-affection diminishes intimacy between you and your partner. Below are simple things you can do for your partner to rekindle the loving feelings and increase both of your oxytocin levels.

Increasing Oxytocin Levels:
- Touch your partner several times a day. A warm, loving hug when you wake up starts the day with an increase in oxytocin production.
- Repeat the hug when leaving for work, returning home at the end of the day and at bedtime. It is suggested that the hug be 15 – 20 seconds long.
- Give your partner a 10-second kiss at least once a day. Look directly and warmly into your partner's eyes.
- While your partner is seated, walk up and give your partner a quick back or neck rub. Massage your partner's feet or scalp while watching TV. Offer to give your partner a full body massage (this can create a significant upsurge in oxytocin).
- Say *"I love you"* frequently.
- Look for opportunities throughout the day to touch your partner:
  - Give your partner a quick pat on the back when passing by.
  - Put an arm around your partner's shoulder when sitting together.
  - Hold hands when walking, giving an occasional light squeeze to emphasize your awareness of the closeness.
- Show interest when your partner talks to you. Stop what you are doing, look your partner in the eye and draw nearer to listen. This action conveys, *"You, and what you say, are important to me."*

Chapter 15

- Talk about a trait you admire or appreciate in your mate while in the presence of friends or family. Everyone wants to be valued and validated, especially in public.
- Validate your mate's loving actions. *"I love it when you help me with the dishes after dinner."* Say *"thank you"* for the little things.
- Smile warmly when you see your partner. When your partner is across the room in a crowd, make eye contact and wink.
- Send your mate a loving message by text, email or write it on a sticky note: *"I love you." "I can't wait to see you." "You are the love of my life." "I am so blessed to have you in my life."*
- Plan a date night where your only focus is on your relationship and having fun.

> **Creating Adventure**
>
> Plan to try a new restaurant on your next date. Newness stimulates and excites the brain. Sit on the same side of the table during the meal. Act like a teenager in love. Rub your partner's leg gently or caress your partner's hand and whisper loving words of affirmation and appreciation.

- Plan to add new experiences with your mate. It has been proven that relationships are strengthened when couples participate in exciting new activities/projects/adventures together. Look at community activities for new ideas to participate in together such as going to a ballgame, art show, concert, book club, canoeing, camping, dancing, etc. Couples often get in a rut when doing the same activities all of the time. When you participate in a new adventure, the activity adds spice to your relationship and increases intimacy.
- Let your partner vent when upset. Simply listen. Don't try to fix the situation or give advice, just give validation that you hear your partner. *"I hear what you are saying." "I can see why you feel ___." "How can I help?"* We all need someone who will be there to stand by us when we are feeling down, tired, discouraged or wronged, without being judgmental or critical. Relationships can be strengthened by simply listening and not jumping in with advice unless you are specifically asked about your opinion.

Understanding Female Sex Drive

- Express appreciation to your partner about something you love doing together: *"I love our morning time together as we drink our coffee." "My favorite thing is the time we spend alone and talking during our daily walk." "Cuddling with you before we go to sleep is always a special time for me."*
- Make positive statements about your life together, *"Isn't it wonderful that we ___?"*

Improving the relationship with your partner is an important part of restoring the sexual relationship. Concentrate on the loving and touching activities listed above to connect meaningfully with your partner. You will find your mood and relationship with your partner soar as your oxytocin level increases.

Chapter 15

Remember

- *Female sex drive is different than the male sex drive. A male has frequent sexual thoughts. Males are driven by high levels of the sex hormone testosterone, which causes them to actively seek sexual encounters. Male sexuality is mostly physically controlled. On the other hand, female sexuality is a complex combination of psychological and physical factors.*

- *The female sex drive is not driven by internal thoughts but is most often accessed by external stimulation of touch and/or words by an acceptable partner.*

- *The hormone oxytocin is the "bonding hormone" that is released by touch. Increased oxytocin levels bring many benefits including a relaxed mood, decreased anxiety, decreased depression and an increase in immunity. Plan to increase your oxytocin levels by increasing touching opportunities with your partner. This will benefit your health and sexual relationship.*

- *If you want to rev up your sex life, mentally determine that you want to engage in a sexual encounter. Then, focus on sexually stimulating thoughts as you prepare yourself and your environment.*

- *Schedule a date night so you can prepare yourself and your environment.*
  - *Prepare in advance by purchasing your favorite love songs, perfume/cologne, candles, silky lingerie, bath oil, vaginal lubricant, silky sheets and massage oil.*
  - *Prepare the room with candles or low lighting, clean sheets and your favorite music. Have sexual lubricant readily available.*
  - *On the night of the date, prepare your mind and body by listening to your music, taking a warm bath, applying your favorite body lotion or perfume and then slipping into your silky lingerie.*
  - *Enjoy the evening!*

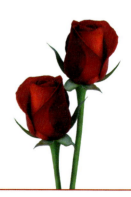

Chapter 16

Increasing Female Sexual Pleasure

In this chapter, we are going to get down to the nuts and bolts of sexuality. We are going to explore the complex issues of creating desire, building excitement and enjoying the sexual act. Sexuality between partners requires a unique blend of psychological and physical components to produce the desired outcome of sexual satisfaction for both partners. Understanding the psychological and physical components required for creating meaningful, enjoyable sexual relations is helpful in restoring your relationship with your partner. Just like baking a cake, if you leave out one ingredient, the outcome can be easily altered. Cancer treatment may have altered some things, but the good news is that there are answers to deal with the changes.

Desire and Romance

Movies and television shows portray romance as occurring without any effort. A touch leads to a kiss, which leads to instant, blazing sex. But, that is simply fiction written into a script. In real life, creating desire and romance does not occur that easily and is vastly different for women and men.

Romance and the creation of desire in a female begin long before the lights are turned off, she is affectionately touched in bed, and the first kiss occurs. Creating desire for a sexual encounter in a female is quite different from creating sexual desire in a male. Women have a strong need for a relationship with a potential sexual partner while males do not have the same degree of need for relationship. Therefore, romance and foreplay to a male and female are totally different. Foreplay to a male may be the first kiss, stroking the body and fondling the genitals after getting into bed. But for a woman, romance and foreplay start much earlier.

Chapter 16

Foreplay, from a woman's perspective, may not even be related to her physical body. Foreplay may start with her perception of value to her sexual partner and is evidenced by actions. A woman's willingness for a sexual encounter can begin with the trash being taken out earlier in the day by her partner, an unexpected phone call to just say *"I love you,"* or the words, *"Let me help you with the dishes."* These interpersonal relationship acts of awareness and caring set the stage for sexual foreplay. The bottom line in sexual readiness is that women desire and need a relationship. The relationship begins long before they are between the sheets. While relationships are important to men, they do not play the same role in sex as they do for women.

It is very important to know the difference between female and male sexual readiness. A woman's desire is like a slow-cooking crock-pot—she gradually and slowly moves toward readiness. On the other hand, male sexual readiness is like a microwave—it is fast and instant. The problem occurs when either partner, male or female, thinks that the other would desire the same type of approach to increase readiness and desire for sexual relationships. I would suggest you share this chapter, along with the tear-out pages beginning on page 197, with your sexual partner. Partner understanding of the information in this chapter can be critical to restoring your sexuality.

Sexually-Stimulating Words

To encourage deeper intimacy, it is important that women and men hear the words that make them feel sexually attracted to one another. The words that sexually stimulate a woman are usually different than the words men find sexually stimulating. The goal is to learn to say words that convey, *"I love you, and I need you,"* by using the words most desired by the partner.

Different Words for Different Genders:
- Women want to hear words about their **attractiveness** and **commitment** from their sexual partner.
- Men want to hear words about their **sexual function** from their sexual partner.

Words That Convey Attractiveness and Commitment To Females:
- *"I am yours forever."*
- *"I never want to be without you."*

Increasing Female Sexual Pleasure

- *"I can't stop thinking about how much I love you."*
- *"You are the greatest thing that ever happened to me."*
- *"Your sweet body fragrance lingers in my mind when we are apart."*
- *"You send shivers up and down my spine when I think of you."*
- *"The feel of your skin is like satin."*
- *"You are a very sensual woman."*
- *"Just seeing you walk across the room excites me."*

Words That Convey Physical or Sexual Approval to Males:
- *"You are the best lover I could ever have."*
- *"You know how to turn me on sexually."*
- *"You are the best in bed."*
- *"Your strong arms cause me to go limp when you hold me."*
- *"I can't resist your warm breath on my neck when you hold me tight."*
- *"You are a perfect '10' in bed."*

Gender defines the words that make the other partner feel more sexually responsive. Even if these phrases or comments do not seem to make sense as being sexually arousing, research has proven them to be so. Try them out and see if they work for your relationship.

Sexually-Stimulating Touch

Gentle, affectionate touching promotes sexual arousal and, eventually, pleasure. Knowing the arousal areas of the body that have the ability to excite and bring pleasure is helpful. The erogenous zones listed below have high concentrations of sensory nerves that add to sexual stimulation and sexual pleasure. Stimulating these areas by touching, licking or kissing can increase arousal and pleasure.

Female Erogenous Zones:
- **Clitoris:** The most erogenous zone in the female body is the clitoris. The clitoris has more nerves than any other part of the female body. Stimulation of the clitoris is the fastest and easiest way to create arousal in a woman. For some women, direct stimulation is not as pleasurable as indirect stimulation to the area surrounding the clitoris. The clitoris extends underneath the skin for about four inches and gentle pressure to this area also increases arousal.

Chapter 16

- **Breasts and Nipples:** The breasts and, especially, the nipples respond to stimulation. The nipples are filled with sensory nerves that stimulate the same region of the brain as the clitoris and vaginal nerves.
- **Cervix:** The cervix is located at the lower end of the uterus and has sensory nerves that respond to pressure stimulation.
- **Mouth and Lips:** Kissing has been found to play a large role in relationship building. Kissing releases oxytocin, the bonding hormone. The lips, mouth and tongue are very sensitive to light touch, temperature or pressure and promote sexual stimulation.
- **Neck:** The back and front of the neck are sensitive to touch. Kissing, licking with the tongue, and warm breathing to the neck can be stimulating to a partner.
- **Ears:** The ears have a large number of nerve ends and are very sensitive to touch. Gentle touching, pulling and licking may be stimulating to a partner.

Male Erogenous Zones:
- **Penis:** The male penis, like the female clitoris, has the highest number of sensory nerves, which are responsive to sexual stimulation.
- **Scrotum:** The male scrotum is one of the most erogenous zones and responds quickly to touch, which leads to sexual arousal.
- **Perineum:** The perineum is the area located between the anus and the scrotum. The nerves in this area also relay sensations of sexual pleasure to the brain when touched or stroked.
- **Neck:** The neck of a male is not as sensitive as the female neck but is still one of the erogenous zones for kissing or licking that increases sexual arousal.
- **Nipples:** As with women, men rank their nipples as highly sensitive to touch. The nipples contain a very high number of sensory nerve receptors. During sexual stimulation, male nipple erection occurs just as it does in females.
- **Mouth and Lips:** The mouth, lips and tongue are all sensitive to touch and kissing and are sexually stimulating.
- **Ears:** The ears have a high number of sensory nerve receptors that respond to touching, kissing or licking and add to male sexual stimulation.

INCREASING FEMALE SEXUAL PLEASURE

Sexually-Stimulating Body Massage

If letter grades were given to sexually-arousing stimulation, sensual massage would score an "A" rating by most women. Sensual body massage prior to sexual intercourse is a guaranteed pleasure stimulator. During the massage, stimulating all the erogenous zones previously listed creates heightened sexual arousal. The guiding rule is slow, tender touch. Don't rush! Sensual massage is extremely helpful for women who have lowered desire due to cancer treatment. It allows a woman to relax and be slowly stimulated to arousal.

Prepare for the massage by purchasing organic oil from your health food store. The best oils for massage include jojoba, hazelnut, apricot kernel, argan, avocado, safflower, rosehip seed, walnut, camelia, coconut, macadamia nut, marula, almond, moringa, grapeseed, sunflower, sesame, mustard, borage oil or mixed oils. All of these are good choices. Experiment with a few to discover which one you prefer.

Sensual Body Massage Tips:
- Select a location for the massage. A hard surface, massage table or bed work well.
- Be sure that the temperature in the room is warm.
- Protect the bed or massage surface with a sheet or towel.
- Turn down the lights, light candles and turn on soft music.
- Use a towel or sheet to cover the body. Keep the body covered during the massage. Only uncover the body part you are massaging while keeping the rest of the body covered.
- Make sure the body is positioned straight on the massage surface to relieve stress and release pressure.
- Warm your hands and the massage oil if needed. Apply the oil to your warm hands and not directly to the skin.
- Begin the massage with the face down. Use gentle stroking or circular motions. Do not use heavy, deep or excessive pressure. Massage the muscles and not the bones, especially near the spine. Massage areas may include the back, neck, head, ears, buttocks, thighs, calves and feet.
- Get feedback; ask if the pressure is too deep or if the temperature of the room is comfortable. When moving to another part of the body, ask if massage in this area is pleasurable. During the massage, pay attention

Chapter 16

to their body tension and relaxation. Relaxed muscle tension, sighing or quiet moaning with pleasure are all signs that the massage is successful. Communication and chemistry between the two of you will make this a success.

- The buttocks are very sensual and respond when a kneading motion is used because of the large amount of soft tissue in the buttocks. Kneading is similar to the way a baker kneads bread. The motion is very simple. First, press the palms down on the muscle tissue; then, push your fingers together into the tissue and move the tissue upward in a lifting motion. Relax the tension of the hands and repeat.

- After the back of the body is fully massaged, the front of the body is massaged while lying face up. Stroke the thighs allowing the stroke to come near the genitals, without directly touching them. Next, move to the chest area.

- Massage the chest area around the breast while leaving the breast tissue for last. After massaging the chest around the breast, start to massage the breasts using gentle pressure around the nipples but avoid massaging the nipples. Nipple erection is a sign of sexual stimulation. When a high level of sexual stimulation occurs, the nipples will reflect the arousal by becoming extremely erect. At the same time, you will notice that body tension noticeably increases, and the pectoralis muscles tighten causing the breast mound to rise as your strokes come near the nipple. Allow this sexual tension to build by continuing to come close to the nipples without touching them. When sexual tension is high, the nipples respond best to very gentle pressure of licking.

- Genital touch is reserved until last. Apply generous amounts of vaginal lubricant to your fingers and use a very light, gentle touch to the external area of the vulva. Move gradually into the folds of the labia. As swelling occurs, begin softly stroking the sides of the clitoris without touching or applying pressure to the clitoris. Many women find direct pressure to the clitoris early in arousal to be uncomfortable. As vaginal congestion increases, attempt to enter the vagina with a lubricated finger. If the vaginal entry is tight, continue external stimulation to increase arousal and then gently reattempt to enter a finger into the vagina.

- Remember, the level of sex hormones determines arousal. Because cancer-treated women are prone to low sex hormone levels, arousal may

Increasing Female Sexual Pleasure

require an extended time for foreplay. Slow and steady sensual touching is one of the best ways to create sexual arousal.

Women love the closeness and attention that massage brings to the relationship. Massage causes a woman to feel special. Sensual massage allows a hormone-deficient woman the time and stimulation needed to reach the sexual excitement stage.

Incorporating sensual massage extends the time of foreplay for the cancer-treated woman while her partner stimulates all of her erogenous tissues. When the massaging partner does not receive reciprocal stimulation during the massage, this delays their sexual arousal. This delay allows the female partner to reach a high level of arousal before penetration is attempted. The full sexual readiness of the female partner before penetration decreases the potential of sexual discomfort or pain. Sensual massage becomes the key to both partners experiencing a satisfying sexual experience.

Female Versus Male Arousal Time

The time needed for sexual arousal is vastly different for males and females. The lack of understanding about this arousal time gap is often the cause of female complaints about painful sex and the inability to experience an orgasm. The quick arousal of the male leads them to believe their partner is experiencing the same level of excitement. This sexual arousal gap contributes to insufficient time for a female to achieve arousal before a male reaches satisfaction.

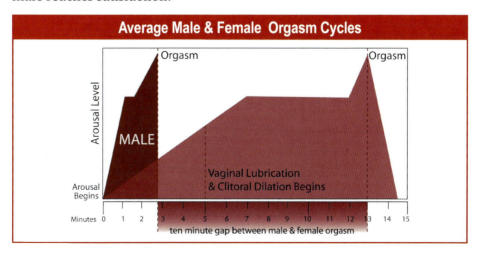

Chapter 16

Arousal time for most males is rapid. From the first sexually stimulated touch, a male can progress to orgasm with ejaculation in about three minutes. The female arousal cycle is much slower. Sexually stimulating touch for a female requires about five minutes for vaginal lubrication and vaginal congestion to occur, creating sexual readiness. At five minutes, the male, without understanding this fact, has no interest in sexual activity, he is satisfied. After female sexual stimulation occurs, it requires approximately ten minutes or more of uninterrupted sexual activity for the average female to reach orgasm.

The sexual arousal time table chart is presented as an average, but the time required varies in individuals. The chart clearly points out the vast difference in time required for arousal and orgasm of males compared to females. It is necessary to understand this difference for mutually satisfying sex to occur. There is a vast difference between the cooking times required for a crock-pot versus a microwave. The same principal applies to males and females in sexual arousal and orgasm. There is a large gap in arousal time.

It is also important to remember that sexual desire, arousal and orgasm are impacted by the reduction of sex hormones after cancer treatment. Sex after cancer treatment changes. What was normal before treatment usually changes, requiring even more time for arousal and orgasm. This requires both partners to understand the changes and learn ways to compensate for them.

Female Sexual Response Cycle

In the l960s, two sexual researchers, Masters and Johnson, researched and described the sexual response cycle for the first time. Their model has undergone modifications over the years, but the basic stages are **(1) desire, (2) excitement, (3) orgasm** and **(4) resolution.**

INCREASING FEMALE SEXUAL PLEASURE

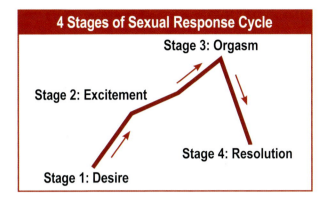

Stage 1: Building Sexual Desire

Desire is described as having interests, thoughts, fantasies and dreams of sexual content. This signifies a state of sexual aliveness or responsiveness that healthy people take for granted.

Sexual Thoughts and Fantasies

- 88% reported having sexual thoughts and fantasies **before** treatment began
- 32% reported having sexual thoughts and fantasies **during** treatment
- 41% reported having sexual thoughts and fantasies **one year after** treatment completion

— *EduCare Focus Group Data*

Desire is governed by both physical and psychological influences. Read through the list of impacting factors that block desire and see if you can identify any issue(s) that you may be experiencing.

Psychological Issues Blocking Desire:

- High levels of stress
- Personal perception of femininity
- Perceived lack of support from sexual partner
- Perceived partner sexual attraction after cancer treatment
- Low personal body image due to surgical changes or weight gain
- Fears
- Chronic anxiety
- Chronic depression

Physiological Issues Blocking Desire:

- Fatigue
- Body pain
- Painful intercourse
- Urinary incontinence

Chapter 16

Reducing the Potential for Painful Intercourse

The majority of women reading this book will deal with vaginal dryness. If vaginal dryness is not treated, it will lead to painful intercourse. If you were premenopausal at diagnosis, you may not have experienced a lack of vaginal lubrication before treatment. The problem of vaginal dryness may be new to you and your partner.

Often, partners do not understand the need for vaginal lubricants. They may not understand that cancer treatment has caused a woman to be unable to lubricate naturally after sexual stimulation. Partners often associate vaginal wetness as a response to their sexual stimulation. When vaginal wetness is absent after foreplay, they may, incorrectly, believe their partner is no longer sexually interested in them. It is necessary to have a mutual understanding of why a lubricant is now needed. Vaginal dryness was caused by chemotherapy, and a vaginal lubricant is necessary to restore pleasure to your sex life. If you have not already done so, plan to have a discussion with your partner about this change.

If you have not yet re-engaged in a sexual relationship, it is helpful to follow the instructions provided in *Chapter 5: Vaginal Dryness and Painful Intercourse* to treat vaginal dryness before you attempt penetration.

If you have resumed your sexual relationship and experienced painful sex, be assured that the correction of vaginal dryness will reverse the pain you experienced. For women who have not had sex for an extended period of time, the vagina may have narrowed and may also contribute to pain. The use of vaginal dilators can correct this condition. Refer to *Appendix B: Vaginal Dilator Therapy* for additional information.

Removing Communication Road Blocks

Restoring desire often starts with restoring emotional intimacy with your partner. Often, women will avoid all types of physical touch because they are afraid it will lead to intercourse, and they do not feel up to sex. Verbalization of your needs for intimacy without sex is extremely important. When you are struggling with fatigue, it is helpful if you tell your partner about your needs. *"I need to be held tonight, even though I don't feel up to sexual intercourse."*

Increasing Female Sexual Pleasure

Changes in Sexual Functioning Discussion
- 43% of the women reported that their sexual partner brought the subject up first
- 53% of the women reported that they brought the subject up first

— *EduCare Focus Group Data*

If your partner is moving too quickly during the arousal stage, it is key to communicate your needs. *"I need you to spend more time in sexual foreplay so I can better reach sexual arousal."* Honest expression of your needs helps both of you. Expressing what you find stimulating is also helpful. *"I really like it when you ____. It really excites me."*

In addition to verbal expression, you need to address and seek help for your problems of fatigue, vaginal dryness and other side effects of treatment that can impact your sexuality.

Stage 2: Building Excitement

Excitement is the second stage on the sexual arousal chart. Sexual desire leads to a state of sexual excitement. This is the stage when the genitals become engorged, and the vagina secretes a slippery lubricating fluid. The excitement stage is where major interruptions of normal functioning can occur due to the side effects of cancer therapy.

Chemotherapy causes instant menopause and greatly reduces the hormonal levels necessary for vaginal engorgement and lubrication to occur. This reduction lingers long after treatment is over. Because of the low levels of sex hormones, additional stimulation during foreplay is required to reach the excitement phase. Even with stimulation, adequate lubrication may not occur. The use of a vaginal lubricant is necessary to compensate for the lack of natural lubrication.

Sexual Arousal
- 86% reported increased time required for sexual arousal after chemotherapy
- 49% reported diminished nipple sensation after chemotherapy

— *EduCare Focus Group Data*

Chapter 16

It is necessary to be aware of the sensitive role the clitoris plays in sexual stimulation to understand the failure to reach an adequate level of excitement. Along with the increased length of time needed for foreplay, increased stimulation of the clitoris is necessary. Partner or self-stimulation to the clitoris is the best intervention to increase your level of excitement. For women who still find arousal difficult, the addition of sex toys that stimulate the clitoris may be explored. Sex therapists recommend the Eros Clitoral Therapy Device.

The FDA has cleared Eros Therapy as a treatment for low sexual arousal. The Eros device is a small, hand-held apparatus fitted with a small removable, replaceable plastic cup. The cup is applied over the genital area to improve blood flow to the clitoris and genitalia. Eros Therapy is a conditioning routine to restore blood flow to your clitoris and genitalia. Increased blood flow intensifies sensation to the clitoris, which boosts vaginal lubrication while increasing the potential for orgasm. This increases overall sexual satisfaction. Eros Therapy requires no medication, only the application of the device to the genital area.

Users of Eros Therapy report that 75 percent have experienced enhanced sexual satisfaction after use of the recommended therapy protocol. The Eros Therapy device can be ordered directly from the company's website, www.eros-therapy.com, with a doctor's prescription.

Recommendation To Increase Excitement

Dr. Rosemary Basson, a specialist in sexuality, studied the issues of low sexual desire and low sexual arousal. Her recommendation for women with little or **no** sexual desire is to submit to their partner's sexual stimulation (foreplay) **before** they experience any **desire** for sexual activity. Her theory is that partner **stimulation creates desire**. Dr. Basson's sexual arousal chart reverses desire and excitement. She recommends that women who have no desire agree to participate in sexual stimulation with their partner and, after adequate stimulation, desire for sexual activity will be created.

Increasing Female Sexual Pleasure

Participation in sexual stimulation before desire has worked well for chemo-treated women and women who find their desire is all but absent.

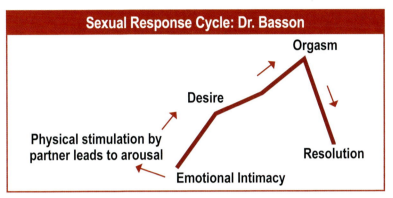

Experiment with your partner. Explain that you want them to sexually stimulate you. It is also recommended that a variety of new stimulation techniques be tried. Monotony causes lack of excitement and is the death of many sex lives. Dr. Basson suggests that couples use sensual massage as an extended foreplay technique. Sensual massage by a partner works on the same concept of stimulation to create desire (*see page 139*). Sex toys can also increase clitoral stimulation; while providing variety in sexual foreplay. A variety of sex toys can be purchased online and delivered to your home with no identifying marks on the package.

Stage 3: Experiencing Orgasm

Orgasm is the third stage of the sexual response cycle. Orgasm is the rhythmic muscular contraction within the female pelvis, which is accompanied by feelings of extreme pleasure. Inability to experience an orgasm after cancer treatment is common. Many times a woman will blame herself for the inability to reach orgasm. Because of this, I want to share with you the focus group data I obtained from chemo-treated cancer patients and their ability to experience orgasm before, during and after treatment.

Chapter 16

Ability to Reach Orgasm			
Orgasm Frequency:	Before Treatment	During Treatment	12 Months After Treatment
Never	1%	24%	10%
Rarely	8%	27%	23%
Occasionally	19%	28%	29%
Most of the Time	55%	16%	30%
All of the Time	17%	5%	9%

— EduCare Focus Group Data

Inability to experience an orgasm is normal for many women during cancer treatment and for some women after treatment.

Stage 4: Experiencing Resolution

Resolution is the fourth stage of the sexual response model. This is the period after a sexual encounter, which includes relaxation of the sexual tension and reduction of the engorgement in the genitals. This should be a time of closeness with the sexual partner and not a reflection on the actual performance. For women having difficulty experiencing an orgasm, it often becomes a time of self-evaluation and remorse over the failure to have an orgasm, which is not helpful. If you find yourself in this category, focus on the beauty of having the ability to participate in a relationship of closeness. Remember that even without having an orgasm, the hormone oxytocin is increased by sexual intercourse.

Benefits of a Sexual Relationship

As previously discussed, oxytocin is commonly referred to as the bonding or cuddle hormone. Oxytocin is produced in both males and females. Because sexual intercourse involves an extended period of hugging and touching, levels of oxytocin greatly increase even if orgasm is not experienced. After intercourse, increased oxytocin causes you to feel relaxed and calm and experience a feeling of closeness toward your partner. Participating in sexual intercourse has many positive benefits for you and your partner, even if you do not have an orgasm. During this time of resolution, enjoy the sense of calm and closeness with your partner without self-judgment.

INCREASING FEMALE SEXUAL PLEASURE

Dr. Basson commented on the lack of orgasm by saying, *"Sexual satisfaction does not necessarily mean that a woman has to have an orgasm. For many women, the feelings of closeness and intimacy and the knowledge that one's partner may have achieved an orgasm may be enough to bring sexual satisfaction to the encounter."*

Advanced "Between the Sheets" Information

For those of you that would like to continue a more in-depth exploration of "between the sheets" sexuality, I highly recommend the book, *Pleasure: A Woman's Guide to Getting the Sex You Want, Need and Deserve*, by Dr. Hilda Hutcherson. Her book clearly explains sexuality questions in understandable terms. Graphically illustrated, the book will help you expand your journey of restoring your sex life with your partner.

Dr. Hutcherson, MD, an obstetrician and gynecologist, is a co-director of the New York Center for Women's Sexual Health at Columbia Presbyterian Medical Center, and an assistant profession of Obstetrics and Gynecology at Columbia University's College of Physicians and Surgeons.

Chapter 16

Remember

- *Good sex is a combination of physical and psychological components that cannot be ignored. Any identified blocks to restoring your sex life must be addressed.*

- *Creating romance that leads to sexual desire is vastly different for women and men. Women have a deep desire for relationship. When relationship is ignored, females have problems creating sexual desire.*

- *Words that create intimacy are important to a sexual relationship. Women like to hear words that convey their attractiveness and commitment from their partner. Men like to hear words conveying approval of their physical and sexual function.*

- *For most females, sensual body massage scores an "A" in pleasure. It allows all female erogenous zones to be gently touched, which slowly increases sexual arousal. Sensual massage allows the female time to gradually reach full arousal. It equalizes the playing field for the sexual arousal time differences between male and female partners.*

- *Touch is an important component of sexual arousal. The female clitoris is the most erogenous zone in the female body. Nipples for some women are extremely sensitive to touch. The clitoris and nipples require gentle, soft touch to respond initially.*

- *Desire, excitement and orgasm had been outlined as the pathway to sexual pleasure. For females with low natural sexual desire, the pathway has changed. It is recommended that females with low or no desire submit to the physical, sexual stimulation by their partner first to create desire. It is after physical stimulation that a woman first experiences desire, which leads to full arousal.*

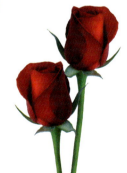

INCREASING FEMALE SEXUAL PLEASURE

Remember

- *It is essential to remember that participating in intercourse increases the release of the hormone, oxytocin, the "feel good" hormone, which is released with or without orgasm. Oxytocin causes you to feel relaxed, calm and closer to your partner.*

- *Regular, sexual excitement and sexual intercourse are recommended to increase blood flow to the vaginal area to heal or prevent dry, damaged tissues and prevent narrowing to the vagina, called vaginal stenosis. Sexual activity also creates a bond between you and your partner, creating psychological connectedness. Participating in sexual activity is good for the mind and the body.*

- *Give yourself the gift of good sex by planning time and saving energy to focus your mind on the joy of human connectedness— the joy of being alive and in relationship with one another. This is the true joy of survivorship.*

Chapter 17

Desire-Enhancing Medications and Supplements

Throughout this book, we have addressed many physical and psychological factors that impact sexuality. Addressing issues, such as vaginal dryness, pain, relationship issues and depression, is necessary before considering physical enhancement medication and supplements. In this chapter, we are going to discuss medication and supplements that have been effective in enhancing desire.

Medication to Increase Desire

Addyi® (flibanserin) is the first FDA approved (August 2015) non-hormonal medication for the treatment of female hypoactive sexual desire disorder (HSDD). Addyi® was first developed as an antidepressant. It adjusts brain chemistry by altering the balance of dopamine and norepinephrine (responsible for sexual excitement) and decreasing levels of serotonin. After clinical studies reported an increased level of desire, it was then marketed as a desire-enhancing drug.

Addyi's® major reported side effects include fainting, nausea, sleepiness, sedation and fatigue. Alcohol should be avoided during treatment. The monthly cost of treatment is approximately $800 and is usually not covered by insurance.

Three clinical studies reported that about ten percent of patients reported improvement in satisfying sexual events and sexual desire. Another study of 2,400 patients reported that Addyi® increased the number of satisfying sexual events by an additional 0.5 – 1 per month compared to placebo. Addyi® has not been shown to enhance sexual performance, only desire.

Chapter 17

Testosterone Therapy

As discussed in an earlier chapter, testosterone is a predominately male hormone, which is associated with sexual desire, arousal and orgasm. Testosterone is also naturally found in much lower levels in females. Testosterone facilitates the female sexual response through increased blood flow to the vagina and clitoris, which causes enhanced engorgement, increased sensation and increased lubrication. Research has shown that testosterone therapy can increase sex drive and can also be a remedy for other sexual problems associated with female menopausal symptoms.

Testosterone preparations are not currently approved by the FDA for use in women. If testosterone is prescribed, it is for off-label use (not approved for the specific condition). Doctors who prescribe testosterone therapy will test blood levels before beginning supplementation and will regularly monitor them to make sure supplemented testosterone levels remain within the therapeutic range. Patients are also monitored for an increase in masculine side-effects such as deepening of the voice, excessive hair growth on face and body, increased size of the clitoris, acne and oily skin.

Most compounded testosterone replacement is made from plant-based sources (bio-identical), which are chemically identical to what the body naturally produces. Testosterone therapy comes in many forms, such as creams, gels, patches, implanted pellets, pills, sublingual (under the tongue) tablets, lozenges or drops.

One of the fears expressed regarding testosterone therapy for estrogen receptor-positive breast cancer patients has been the conversion of testosterone to estradiol. The concern has been that testosterone would increase estradiol levels and negate the effect of the aromatase inhibitor on the reduction of breast cancer recurrence. Recently, two clinical studies were conducted of compounded vaginal testosterone cream that was administered for four weeks to women taking an aromatase inhibitor. The study revealed that patients experienced an increase in sexual arousal, lubrication, orgasm frequency and overall sexual satisfaction while they experienced a reduction of vaginal dryness and vaginal pain. These study results showed that estradiol and testosterone levels remained within safe menopausal levels while decreasing vaginal atrophy and increasing sexual satisfaction.

Desire-Enhancing Medications and Supplements

Because the long-term safety of testosterone therapy for women is unknown, some doctors are hesitant to recommend it; while other doctors feel confident in prescribing it based on current studies. Testosterone therapy is most often prescribed by physicians who specialize in hormone replacement therapy. If you feel that this is a therapy you would like to investigate, you can contact a local compounding pharmacist and ask for a list of doctors in your area who specialize in hormone therapy replacement.

Blood Flow Enhancement Supplements

In this section, we will discuss supplements that enhance blood to flow to the genitals. You may wish to discuss this list with your healthcare provider to determine whether you have any restrictions that would prevent you from trying any of these supplements. *Word of caution: If vaginal dryness has not been corrected, topical enhancing products may increase burning and irritation.*

L-arginine

L-arginine is an amino acid that is found naturally in the body and plays a role in increasing immunity. When it is taken at high levels as a supplement, it increases nitric oxide in the body. Increased levels of nitric oxide cause blood vessels to dilate and allow more blood to flow into them. When blood flow is increased in the genitals, sexual arousal and sensitivity are increased. L-arginine works in a way similar to the way Viagra® works for men, by increasing blood flow. Up to 5 grams a day may be needed to increase desire.

ArginMax®

ArginMax® is a combination of sexual enhancing compounds known to increase blood flow by improving circulation. ArginMax® contains l-arginine as the main ingredient. It also contains Korean Ginseng, Ginkgo biloba, vitamins and minerals. ArginMax® is taken in pill form and does not require a prescription. It comes in two formulations, one designed for women and one designed for men. Two clinical studies have found that ArginMax® improved sexual function in menopausal women.

Ginkgo Biloba

Ginkgo biloba has been used in traditional Chinese medicine for thousands of years. It has been used to boost mental power and increase memory in Alzheimer's patients. It is also used to treat asthma, fatigue and sexual

Chapter 17

dysfunction. Ginkgo biloba increases nitric oxide in the body, which increases blood flow. Ginkgo biloba is thought to also help with sexual dysfunction caused by SSRI (selective serotonin reuptake inhibitor) anti-depressants. Ginkgo biloba is an ingredient found in many sexual enhancing supplements, but it may be taken alone.

Ginseng

Ginseng is a herb that works to increase nitric oxide, which increases blood flow. It also increases energy and improves mood. Ginseng is also used in combination with other compounds to enhance sexual function.

Yohimbe

Yohimbe is a chemical derived from the bark of a tree native to Africa. It is used to increase sexual arousal and excitement. It may also be used for sexual problems caused by an SSRI anti-depressant, and for general sexual problems in both men and women. Other uses for Yohimbe include athletic performance, weight loss, fatigue reduction, diabetic nerve pain and depression.

Yohimbe contains a chemical called yohimbine, which can increase blood flow and nerve impulses to the penis or vagina. It is recommended that you look carefully at the ingredients listed on the bottle label to be sure that the active ingredient is "yohimbine" or "yohimbine hydrochloride." There are other products that have similar names but are not the authentic yohimbine.

Zestra®

Zestra® is a blend of botanical oils and extracts designed to increase female sexual desire by increasing blood flow when applied to the female genitals. Ingredients include borage seed oil, evening primrose oil, angelica extract, coleus extract, Vitamin C and Vitamin E. Zestra® can be purchased over-the-counter in the pharmacy section.

Horny Goat Weed

Horny goat weed is an herb that has been used in Chinese medicine for years. In Chinese medicine, it is labeled as "yin yang huo." Horny goat weed contains an enzyme that helps increase blood flow to the genitals and may improve sexual function.

Desire-Enhancing Medications and Supplements

Vitamin B Complex
Vitamin B complex is available over-the-counter in the pharmacy vitamin section. Vitamin B complex increases energy and decreases depression. B vitamins are essential to convert carbohydrates into usable energy. B vitamins are water soluble and do not accumulate and store in the body, which means they need to be taken daily to maintain adequate levels. Look for the "complex" formula when purchasing Vitamin B. When taking Vitamin B complex, you will find that your urine becomes bright yellow in color. Vitamin B complex is a "must-have" to ensure high levels of energy and an increased mood. A higher level of energy and attitude can provide the spark needed for sexual activity.

Scream Cream
Scream Cream is a topical cream that has been proven to stimulate blood flow to the female genital area. It increases sensitivity and improves the frequency and intensity of orgasms. The cream is applied directly to the clitoris 30 minutes prior to an anticipated sexual encounter. Scream Cream effects last from 30 minutes to 2 hours. The cream causes a local effect only and is not absorbed systemically.

Scream Cream Ingredients
- L-arginine 15mg
- Pentoxifylline 12.5mg
- Aminophylline 7.5mg
- Sildenafil Citrate 2.5mg
- Isosorbide Dinitrate 0.625 mg
- Ergoloid Mesylate 0.123mg
- Testosterone 0.25mg

Scream Cream contains a combination of prescription and non-prescription components described as blood flow enhancers and vasodilators (blood vessel relaxants). L-arginine is one of the main ingredients. The ingredients are all approved by the FDA. The formulation can be custom-tailored to each individual's needs at the request of her healthcare provider. A prescription from your healthcare provider is required and is filled by a compounding pharmacy.

Making Medication and Therapy Decisions
Making a decision about medications, therapies and treatments is often difficult for patients, especially when some recommendations may not be considered mainstream. This is when you, as the patient, have to do research and come to your own conclusion about the risk and benefit ratio

Chapter 17

for yourself. The determining factor has to be what is important to your quality of life. Every medication and therapy comes with both risks and benefits. Even aspirin, a drug that has been widely used since 1899, comes with a list of precautions and potential risks. Yet, we know that there are many positive benefits for patients who need the medication. The decision to take aspirin is an example of a risk/benefit decision.

While making your decision, you have to be aware that there are negative risks with any medication or therapy, but there are also positive benefits. The question you need to ask yourself is, *"Will the benefit I receive outweigh the potential risks?"* This question is one that only you can answer.

Rebuilding your life involves deciding what is right for you. Sometimes, you may have to change healthcare providers to find one that takes your decision-making into consideration and honors your desire to make an informed decision regarding your quality of life. Remember, this is your life; you need to be able to decide what risks are acceptable to you.

DESIRE-ENHANCING MEDICATIONS AND SUPPLEMENTS

Remember

- *Blood flow to the genitals is essential for sexual arousal. Chemotherapy and anti-hormonal therapy like tamoxifen or aromatase inhibitors cause the hormone levels of estrogen and testosterone to be decreased. Lower hormonal levels decrease sexual arousal.*

- *Supplements that increase nitric oxide in the body promote increased blood flow to the genitals, which increases arousal and orgasm intensity.*

- *Vitamin B complex increases energy levels and elevates mood. Daily dosing is necessary because it does not store in the body.*

- *Ask your healthcare provider if you have any restrictions that would prevent you from trying any of the supplements discussed in this chapter.*

Chapter 18

Reclaiming Your Life After Cancer

This chapter will discuss "clearing the deck" for good health. This topic is directly related to your future health and to restoring your sexual intimacy. In the opening chapter of this book, we discussed how an enjoyable sex life is dependent on many influencing factors. Ignoring any one of these factors can sabotage your success for having the best sexual relationship possible. Reclaiming your sex life begins with "clearing the deck" of emotional and physical barriers.

We all know the joy we feel after we finish spring cleaning our house or packing the last box when preparing for a move. We eliminate accumulated junk, clean and reorder our living environment. No one looks forward to spring cleaning or moving because it is hard work. Decisions about what we want to keep or what we want to get rid of often create an internal emotional struggle, which creates stress. We find that we want to keep everything. These things are often taking over our lives and require space and attention. However, after the tough decisions are made, we can sit back and enjoy the rewards of a newly ordered environment.

The same principle is often in place in our personal lives. Our lives accumulate a lot of junk—obligations, activities, personal involvements and commitments. These things clutter our lives and take our time. They leave us little time and energy for ourselves. We come to the end of a day and find that there is no "me" time left after we fulfill all of our obligations. The reality is, our life is on the back burner. We are not a priority on our own schedule. We often find that our lives have been hijacked by the agendas of other people. When we reflect on what is consuming our time, we see that activities that benefit others consume many of our hours, days and weeks. Serving others is a wonderful thing, but not when it comes at

Chapter 18

the sacrifice of your health and happiness. At this point in your life, this is not helpful. This should be a time to concentrate on your physical and emotional recovery. After cancer treatment is the perfect time to spring clean and "clear the deck" to reclaim your life.

I highly recommend that you pause and look closely at your life to determine what is consuming your time. Scrutinize all activities and relationships to determine what value each one brings to your life and health. Often, this scrutiny reveals a life filled with many activities and relationships that are not contributing to your personal health or happiness. After honest evaluation, it is time to spring clean your life.

Having had a cancer diagnosis gives you permission to reclaim your life. It is a call to make tough decisions to rid your life of obligations and activities that do not contribute to your future health. This decision is a gift that only you can give yourself. No one else will ever suggest that it is time for you to give up an activity that benefits them. Seize this opportunity. Clean out the junk you have accumulated over the years. Return the junk that has been placed on your plate by other people and allow them to care for it themselves. The enemy of these decisions is thoughts of, *"But I have always …"* or *"I feel responsible for …"*. Remember, you are now in a new era of life. You are in a place where you need all of your energy to concentrate on building health and immunity. The decision to move forward and build a better life is one that only you can make.

Out of My Cancer Came Good

"I am a seamstress. For years, people would call me with their last-minute emergencies of needing a dress made or needing alterations for a special occasion. I would always say 'yes,' and then I would be required to burn the midnight oil to meet their needs. Now that I have had cancer, I simply say, 'I am so sorry. I have cancer, and I can't do this now even though I would like to.' I can't believe that I have found the courage to speak up. My newfound courage to take care of myself has been the best thing about having cancer. I found that I can say 'no' and take care of myself. Wow! I wish I had done this years ago."

— Patient, EduCare Focus Group

Reclaiming Your Life After Cancer

Suggestions for Reclaiming Your Life After Cancer

- Clean up your life by removing unproductive activities and replacing them with activities that promote your health and well-being. Ask yourself these questions: *"Is this something I want to do? Is this contributing to my happiness? Is this contributing to building my future health?"* If the answer to any of these questions is "no", the activity needs to be closely reviewed to see if it may need to be eliminated from your schedule.

- Determine what is causing you stress. Only you can determine your stressors. What causes one person stress may be another person's stress reducer. List your stressors and determine how you can change or eliminate as many as possible from your life.

- Evaluate your relationships. Relationships can be some of the most stress-producing things in our lives. If a relationship is a stressor to you, reevaluate it. Some relationships cannot be abandoned, but they can be given new guidelines or boundaries. You can learn to set boundaries so the relationship is a win-win situation. If you are not sure how to set a boundary, I highly suggest the book *Boundaries*, by Dr. Cloud and Dr. Townsend. This book has changed the lives of millions of people by teaching them how to deal effectively with relationships. This is one of the greatest principles in their book: *"If you are working harder on the relationship than the other person (giving more and doing more to sustain it), you probably don't need the relationship."* Adult relationships need to be mutually beneficial. If you have a relationship where you are providing the majority of the time, energy or financial funding with no reciprocation from the other person, examine it closely.

- Another area for evaluation is abuse. If you are the victim of verbal or physical abuse, it is time for you to speak up and stand up. Many people are the victims of verbal abuse, which only leaves evidence in one's spirit. It takes courage and support to confront either type of abuse. The first step is to seek help from a professional (social worker, psychologist, professional counselor or psychiatrist) to develop skills to deal with the abuse. They can help you identify a community of supportive people who will work with you to teach you how to protect yourself.

- Work on adding the word "no" to your vocabulary. Learn to smile and say, *"Thank you for asking. I would love to, but I have to say NO at this time."* No other explanation is needed. Absolutely NO guilt needs to be

Chapter 18

accepted either! This is your life. Other people will quickly fill up your time with their agenda if you are not prepared to decline their offer to use your time and talents for their benefit.

- Adopt a healthy lifestyle of diet and exercise. The benefits produce future health, energy, productivity and happiness. Sleep is not a luxury; it is an essential component of good health. Be sure that your new life plan includes time to get adequate sleep.
- Give up your desire to be right or your attempt to be perfect. Having to be right all of the time will steal your energy, happiness and eventually your health. It is a high price to pay. Accept that you are human, and mistakes happen. Let things go. Physical and emotional health are of much higher personal value than having to be right or perfect.
- Realize the high price of arguments and anger on your immunity and health. Every time we get angry, upset or stressed, our body responds by secreting the hormone cortisol. Cortisol has a well-documented, weakening effect on the body's immune response. Cortisol blocks T-lymphocyte cells (T-cells) which are an essential component of cell-mediated immunity. These are the cells that protect our body from disease and cancer. Anger, bitterness and stress all have a direct impact on our future health. Stop the avoidable release of the stress hormone cortisol. Avoid unnecessary stress by avoiding unnecessary conflict.
- Take time throughout the day to relax and recharge your batteries. Plan mini self-care breaks throughout the day. Take a walk. Listen to your favorite music. Hold a baby. Play with a young child. Take a warm bath. Smile at a stranger. Stop to speak to an older person. Read something inspirational. Make a gratefulness list. Volunteer. Tell someone how much they mean to you. Write an encouraging note to someone. These small mini-breaks will bring you joy and help to quiet your spirit. A quiet, joyful spirit creates physical immunity, which governs health.
- Laughter is often rare or forgotten in the midst of dealing with a cancer diagnosis and undergoing treatment. During treatment, there is little time or reason to laugh. But, now that the crisis has passed, it is time to identify future health-building activities, and laughter is one of those. Laughter is a proven health-building activity. It lowers blood pressure, reduces stress hormones in the body, boosts T-cells that increase immunity, and releases endorphins that decrease pain and increase

mood. Find what makes you laugh and add it to your life. Watching funny movies is a great way to add laughter to your life.

- To reduce your stress, take advantage of the benefits of a supportive relationship. An intimate relationship, which provides support, is a barrier against distress and can lessen the feelings of inadequacy when coping with life situations. Avoiding, or limiting, time with negative people and seeking relationships and activities where you are valued is helpful to your emotional and physical health. *"Go where you are celebrated and not just tolerated"* is a freeing and health-building life principle.
- Remind yourself that taking quality time to work on restoring your sexual relationship with your partner is health-producing. Mutually enjoyable sexual encounters increase the bonding between you and your partner and promotes the release of the hormone oxytocin. Oxytocin relaxes the body and decreases your level of stress hormones, primarily cortisol, which increases your immunity and lowers your blood pressure.

Your cancer diagnosis has given you the opportunity to reexamine your life and make changes that only you can make. Cancer is an invitation to take charge of your future health and happiness. Don't let this opportunity pass you by. You deserve it.

Work Had Hijacked My Life

"My cancer diagnosis came as a negative surprise that changed me. Cancer changed the way I now live my life and how I think about my future. After I returned home from surgery and was recuperating, I realized my work/life balance was NOT in balance. As a single career woman, I had let my work take over my life. I recognized that in order to recover physically and emotionally, I needed to change the balance.

I reduced my work hours to from 60 – 70 hours per week to 40 – 50, which has had a very positive impact on my life. I realized that I needed to make more time for me, not in a selfish way, but in an empowering way; I needed to rebuild my health and my life. I now use that time for self-care and nurturing. Fitness has become a big part of my healing journey."

— Breast Cancer Survivor

Chapter 18

Personal Quality of Life Post-Assessment
Where Do You Stand Today?
Complete the assessment on the following page. Rate your present state or condition in each area using the following scale:

1 = None/Little/Never/Low/No problem
(Does not interfere with quality of life)

3 = Occasional/Minimal/Tolerable
(Moderately interferes with quality of life)

5 = Severe/Very Frequent/High
(Severely interferes with quality of life)

Compare the results of the ***Post-Assessment*** with the results of your ***Pre-Assessment*** on page 18. If you do not see a significant increase in your quality of life after reading this book and implementing recommended strategies and interventions, take this assessment to a healthcare professional.

For physical functioning problems, seek a professional specializing in women's health. For relationship difficulties, seek a psychological counselor, psychologist or psychiatrist for further help.

Continue to seek the help you deserve to restore your quality of life after cancer treatment.

Reclaiming Your Life After Cancer

Personal Quality of Life Assessment: Post-Assessment

Physical Symptoms	Level of Distress
Fatigue	(None) 1 2 3 4 5 (Severe)
Headaches	1 2 3 4 5
Hot Flashes	1 2 3 4 5
Night Sweats	1 2 3 4 5
Anxiety/Nervousness	1 2 3 4 5
Depression	1 2 3 4 5
Insomnia	1 2 3 4 5
Vaginal Dryness	1 2 3 4 5
Painful Intercourse	1 2 3 4 5
Loss of Sexual Libido	1 2 3 4 5
Weight Gain	1 2 3 4 5
Pain	1 2 3 4 5
Urine Leakage	1 2 3 4 5
Relationship Assessment	**Level**
Significant Other	☐ Good ☐ Stressful ☐ Very Stressful
Immediate Family	☐ Good ☐ Stressful ☐ Very Stressful
Close Friends	☐ Good ☐ Stressful ☐ Very Stressful
Social Life	☐ Good ☐ Stressful ☐ Very Stressful
Sexual Assessment	**Level**
Sex Drive (Libido)	☐ Good ☐ Low ☐ Very Low
Orgasm Ability	☐ Always ☐ Occasional ☐ Never
Body Image Assessment	**Level**
Physical Appearance	☐ Good ☐ Acceptable ☐ Unacceptable
Weight	☐ Good ☐ Acceptable ☐ Unacceptable
Overall Assessment	**Level**
Quality of Life: Physical	(Good) 1 2 3 4 5 (Poor)
Quality of Life: Psychological	1 2 3 4 5
Quality of Life: Relational	1 2 3 4 5

Chapter 18

"To the problems of your life, you are the only solution."

— Jo Coudert, Author

"The most beautiful people we have known are those who have known defeat, known suffering, known struggle, known loss and have found their way out of the depths. These persons have an appreciation, a sensitivity, and an understanding of life that fills them with compassion, gentleness, and a deep loving concern. Beautiful people do not just happen."

— Elizabeth Kubler-Ross, Psychiatrist

"If you're going through hell, keep going."

— Winston Churchill

"My cancer diagnosis changed my life. I am grateful for every new, healthy day I have. It helped me prioritize my life."

— Olivia Newton-John, Actress

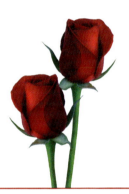

"Cancer is not what I thought it was—a death sentence. It was rather a life sentence; it pushed me to learn how to LIVE my life."

— Patient, EduCare Focus Group

A Final Word

Hopefully, in this book you have found some insights that have assisted you in reducing the lingering side effects of cancer treatment that were interfering with your quality of life, especially your sex life. As we stated at the beginning of this book, no woman regrets seeking and receiving treatment for a potentially life-threatening disease; they are grateful for the life-saving treatment. However, women need and deserve help to deal with the treatment side effects to minimize the impact on their daily quality of life.

Cancer creates a sisterhood of women who share a common journey with similar challenges. On this journey, the experiences of others who have traveled ahead of you offer the greatest encouragement. It is from their sharing of experiences that others who travel behind can benefit and avoid many of the same roadblocks. "Forewarned is forearmed" allows others to anticipate what to expect and to prepare adequately. Being forewarned reduces the shock and the feeling of being alone when confronted by a challenge, which lessens the overall emotional and physical impact on a patient.

Now that you understand that changes in sexuality after cancer treatment are normal for most women, you can help other women. My desire is that you will share the information you have learned with your fellow cancer journeyers. You can help them avoid some of the struggles you have gone through.

It has been my privilege to share this journey of restoring your sexual functioning after cancer treatment.

Good Health To You,

Judy

Appendix and Reference

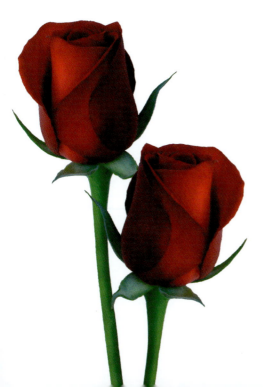

Appendix A

Comparison of Breast Reconstruction Procedures

	Tissue Expander and Implant
Procedure	■ Expander placed under muscle to gradually stretch ■ Second surgery for fixed-volume implant
Advantages	■ Shorter surgical and recovery time compared to autologous
Disadvantages	■ No immediate breast mound ■ Expander requires multiple saline fillings (4 - 6 months) ■ 2nd surgery for implant placement ■ Future replacement in 10 – 15 years ■ Potential risks: capsular contracture, leakage or rupture
Recommended	■ Medium size breast (400 – 800 cc) ■ Bilateral reconstruction
Not Recommended	■ Future radiation therapy planned

	Fixed-Volume Implant Only (Saline or Silicone)
Procedure	■ Fixed-volume implant placed at surgery
Advantages	■ Immediate breast mound ■ Shorter surgical time compared to autologous ■ One-step procedure
Disadvantages	■ Future replacement in 10 – 15 years ■ MRI surveillance; 3 years after placement, then every 2 years ■ Potential risks: capsular contracture, leakage or rupture
Recommended	■ Bilateral reconstruction ■ Tight skin from previous radiation therapy
Not Recommended	■ Future radiation therapy planned

APPENDIX A

DIEP (Deep Inferior Epigastric Perforator)

Procedure	- Autologous abdominal: skin and fat - Blood supply cut (free flap)
Advantages	- Immediate breast mound - Shorter recovery than pedicle TRAM - Abdominal muscle not moved - Decreases abdominal weakness or hernia risk over TRAM - Improves abdominal contour
Disadvantages	- Scar on abdomen - Longer surgical time than pedicle TRAM - Requires microsurgery - Potential risks: seroma, flap necrosis
Recommended	- Mastectomy - Women with extra abdominal fat
Not Recommended	- Previous abdominal scarring from surgery or liposuction - Certain physical conditions - Smokers - Extremely thin women (limited body fat)

TRAM Flap
(Transverse Rectus Abdominis Myocutaneous)

Procedure	- Autologous abdominal (stomach): skin, fat and muscle tunnelled under skin - Blood supply **not** cut (pedicle flap)
Advantages	- Immediate breast mound - Does not require microsurgery - "Tummy tuck"; improves abdomen contour
Disadvantages	- Muscle cut and included with moved tissue - Scar on abdomen - Longer surgery than implant - Difficulty standing up straight for several days - 6 - 8 weeks of recovery - Abdominal weakness - Potential risks: seroma, flap necrosis, abdominal wall hernia
Recommended	- Mastectomy - Women with extra abdominal fat
Not Recommended	- Previous abdominal scarring from surgery or liposuction - Certain physical conditions - Smokers

Breast Reconstruction Procedures

Latissimus Dorsi Flap

Procedure	■ Autologous back: skin, fat and muscle tunnelled under skin ■ Blood supply **not** cut (pedicle flap)
Advantages	■ Immediate breast mound ■ Does not require microsurgery
Disadvantages	■ Small donor scar on back ■ Shoulder weakness ■ Potential risks: seroma, flap necrosis risk
Recommended	■ Small to medium size breast (200 – 600 cc) ■ Tight skin from radiation therapy ■ Future radiation therapy planned
Not Recommended	■ Extremely thin (limited body fat)

TAP (Thoracodorsal Artery Perforator)

Procedure	■ Autologous back: skin and fat
Advantages	■ Immediate breast mound ■ Does not require microsurgery ■ No muscle cut or moved
Disadvantages	■ Small donor scar on back ■ Potential risks: seroma, flap necrosis
Recommended	■ Small to medium sized breast (200 – 600 cc) ■ Tight skin from radiation therapy ■ Future radiation therapy planned
Not Recommended	■ Extremely thin (limited body fat)

Appendix A

IGAP (Inferior Gluteal Artery Perforator)

Procedure	■ Autologous buttock: skin and fat ■ Blood supply cut (free flap)
Advantages	■ Immediate breast mound ■ Most women have adequate fatty tissue
Disadvantages	■ Scar at donor site ■ Requires microsurgery ■ Potential risks: seroma, flap necrosis
Recommended	■ Mastectomy ■ Women with additional buttock fat ■ Women who are not candidates for abdominal procedures
Not Recommended	■ Smokers ■ Extremely thin women (limited body fat)

SGAP (Superior Gluteal Artery Perforator)

Procedure	■ Autologous buttock: skin and fat ■ Blood supply cut (free flap)
Advantages	■ Immediate breast mound ■ Most women have adequate fatty tissue ■ No muscle cut or moved ■ Scar hidden by underwear
Disadvantages	■ Scar at donor site ■ Requires microsurgery ■ Potential risks: seroma, flap necrosis
Recommended	■ Mastectomy ■ Women with additional buttock fat ■ Women that are not candidates for abdominal procedures
Not Recommended	■ Smokers ■ Extremely thin women (limited body fat)

Breast Reconstruction Procedures

TUG (Transverse Upper Gracilis)

Procedure	- Autologous thigh: skin, fat and small amount of muscle - Blood supply cut (free flap)
Advantages	- Immediate breast mound - Thigh tissue rarely damaged from previous surgeries
Disadvantages	- Scar at donor site - Requires microsurgery - Potential risks: seroma, flap necrosis
Recommended	- Bilateral mastectomy; bilateral reconstruction - Women that are not candidates for abdominal procedures
Not Recommended	- Smokers - Certain medical conditions

PAP (Profunda Artery Perforator)

Procedure	- Autologous thigh: skin and fat - Blood supply cut (free flap)
Advantages	- Immediate breast mound - Thigh tissue rarely damaged from previous surgeries
Disadvantages	- Scar at donor site - Requires microsurgery - Potential risks: seroma, flap necrosis
Recommended	- Bilateral mastectomy; bilateral reconstruction - Women that are not candidates for abdominal procedures
Not Recommended	- Smokers - Certain medical conditions

Appendix B

Vaginal Dilator Therapy

As discussed in *Chapter 5: Vaginal Dryness and Painful Intercourse*, menopause or chemotherapy treatment causes a great reduction in the hormone estrogen. Lack of estrogen causes changes in the vagina. One condition is vaginal stenosis. The narrowing of the vaginal canal can lead to painful intercourse. Vaginal dilators are designed to gradually stretch and restore the size of your vagina, allowing you to once again have vaginal sex or a vaginal exam without experiencing pain.

Vaginal dilators are available for purchase online. It is suggested that you purchase a set with graduated (increasing) sizes. This will allow you to begin with a size that is not painful and gradually increase the size until you have stretched the vaginal canal to its previous size.

Before starting dilator therapy, allow your healthcare provider to perform a thorough vaginal exam to rule out any other vaginal problems. During this exam, your physician can tell you the appropriate size of dilator to begin your therapy.

Using a Vaginal Dilator:
- Select a comfortable location to perform dilator therapy. Most women find their bedroom works well.
- Gather the items you will need: your set of dilators, a lubricant, a small mirror and a towel to lie on.
- While lying on your back, pull your knees up to a 45-degree angle. Place your feet shoulder width apart on the bed.
- Perform a set of Kegel exercises. *(See page 61.)*
- Apply the lubricant to the opening of your vagina. Using one finger, apply lubricant to the inside of the vagina.
- Select the dilator size recommended by your physician and generously apply a lubricant to it.

Appendix B

- Holding the dilator with your dominant hand, slowly insert the round end of the dilator into your vagina using a slightly upward angle. (Never use a downward angle.)
- Using gentle pressure, insert the dilator until you feel slight discomfort or muscle tension; then stop. The goal is for the dilator to feel snug, but not painful. Never force the dilator.
- If you find that the dilator size you selected is very easy to insert, select the next size up. The goal is to find one that meets with some resistance when inserting.
- With the dilator in place, perform another set of Kegel exercises to relax your pelvic floor muscles; then insert the dilator a little further. If it is still difficult to insert further, take five deep breaths and exhale forcefully. Attempt to insert the dilator further again. If unable to insert further or if it is painful, simply stop at that point and leave the dilator in place for 5 – 10 minutes.
- Before removing the dilator, gently and slowly push it back and forth 5 to 10 times to stretch the length of your vagina.
- Next, rotate the dilator gently and slowly in wide circles 5 – 10 times to stretch the width of your vagina.
- Remove the dilator from your vagina.
- Wash the dilator in hot, soapy water and dry thoroughly. Store in the container provided by the manufacturer.

After Dilator Therapy:

- It is normal to experience a small amount of bleeding after dilator therapy. Prepare by using a panty liner.
- It is suggested that you urinate after dilator therapy to prevent a urinary tract infection.
- *Warning: Use a dilator to the point of discomfort, but NOT pain. If a significant amount of bleeding occurs (to the degree it soaks a sanitary napkin), contact your healthcare provider.*

Plan to perform dilator therapy every other day. It is recommended that you apply a vaginal moisturizer at least three times a week at bedtime.

Appendix C

Sexuality After Breast Cancer Treatment Focus Group Study

EduCare Inc. conducted 11 national focus groups of women to investigate the impact of breast cancer surgery and chemotherapy on sexual functioning during 2000 and 2001.

Participating Facilities

- Elliott Hospital, Manchester, New Hampshire
- Kettering Medical Center, Dayton, Ohio
- Grant Riverside Methodist Hospital, Columbus, Ohio
- St. Francis Hospital, Indianapolis, Indiana
- Southern Illinois University, Springfield, Illinois
- Don and Sybil Harrington Cancer Center, Amarillo, Texas
- Scripps, San Diego, California
- Northside Hospital, Atlanta, Georgia
- St. Joseph's Women's Hospital, Tampa, Florida
- Lexington Medical Center, Columbia, South Carolina
- Breast Cancer Support Groups, Diana Wall, Las Vegas, Nevada

Area of Country Where Participants Received Treatment:

- Northeast 26%
- Central 17%
- West 25%
- Southeast 14%
- Southwest 18%

Appendix C

Composition of Focus Groups

Number of Participants:
- Number of breast cancer survivors participating in groups ... 126

Age of Participants at Diagnosis:
- 23 - 30 years 3%
- 31 - 35 years 6%
- 36 - 40 years 7%
- 41 - 45 years ..15%
- 46 - 50 years ..27%
- 51 - 55 years ..17%
- 56 - 60 years ..12%
- 61 - 65 years 9%
- 66 and over 4%

Menopausal State at Diagnosis:
- 58% ... Pre-Menopausal
- 24% ... Menopausal
- 18% ... Surgical Menopause

Data Collection Method

- 143 questions were asked of participants in sessions lasting from 2 to 3.5 hours.
- Data was collected by participants using individual hand-held interactive data computer pads.
- Before participants answered each question, a thorough explanation was provided to ensure accurate interpretation of each question.
- Participants were assured all answers were completely anonymous.
- Participants were instructed not to respond to those questions that were not applicable to their situation.
- Participants selected their response and entered their answer into their computer pad.
- Participants were immediately able to see anonymous individual and collective responses of the group on the screen.

Focus Group Study

Focus Group Questions

- Questions were selected to gain basic demographic data and information about the types of cancer treatments received by participants.
- Questions were reviewed by dedicated breast cancer nurses and physicians for appropriateness.
- Main goals of the questions:
  - Define the personal interpretation of various factors that could impact sexual functioning including physical, psychological and interpersonal relationships.
  - Define the impact on quality of life comparing pre-treatment quality of life status to treatment stages including (1) during treatment, (2) six months after treatment completion and (3) one year after treatment completion. Collecting this data was accomplished by the participant assigning a baseline quality of life rating and then comparing the change of this baseline during treatment, six months after and one year after completion of treatment.
  - Define what patient teaching and support by the healthcare team would have been helpful in areas of sexuality.
- Participants were asked to define the impact of the following factors on sexual functioning:
  - Chemotherapy
  - Body image
  - Fatigue
  - Hot flashes
  - Night sweats
  - Insomnia
  - Vaginal dryness
  - Painful intercourse
  - Vaginal infections
  - Mood swings
  - Anxiety and nervousness
  - Depression
  - Anger and aggression
  - Weight gain
  - Hair loss
  - Ability to reach orgasm
- All focus group data was combined and analyzed by computer.
- If a patient had experienced recurrence, she was instructed to answer questions about her first surgical and chemotherapy experience.

Appendix C

Participant Treatment History

Surgery Type:
- 54% ... Lumpectomy
- 46% ... Mastectomy

Lumpectomy: 90% of participants also received radiation therapy.

Mastectomy Patients Reconstruction Decision:
- 46% ... No Reconstruction
- 42% ... Immediate Reconstruction
- 12% ... Delayed Reconstruction

Reconstruction Surgery Selection:
- 39% ... TRAM Flap
- 22% ... Saline Implant
- 19% ... Silicone Implant
- 11% ... Free Flap
- 8% ... Latissimus Dorsi
- 0% ... Autologous & Implant

Reconstruction Timing by Types:
- Saline Implant: .... 14% Immediate .... 33% Delayed
- Silicone Implant: .... 5% Immediate .... 44% Delayed
- TRAM Flap: .... 57% Immediate .... 0% Delayed
- Latissimus Dorsi: .... 10% Immediate .... 11% Delayed
- Free Flap: .... 14% Immediate .... 11% Delayed

Chemotherapy Treatment Protocols:
- 51% ... Adriamycin/Cytoxan
- 32% ... Adriamycin/Taxol/Taxotere
- 10% ... CMF
- 4% .... Didn't Know
- 3% ..... Other

Cessation of Menstrual Period During Treatment:
- 82% ... Cessation of Period
- 18% ... Continuing or Irregular Periods

Chemotherapy Cessation of Periods:
- 91% ... Adriamycin/Taxol/Taxotere
- 83% ... CMF
- 79% ... Adriamycin/Cytoxan

Focus Group Study

Participant Education Data

Surgical Options Patient Education:
- 80% ... Reported that they felt that their physicians/nurses explained options so that they were able to make the surgical decisions that were best for them
- 11% ... Reported that they somewhat understood options after receiving education
- 9% .... Reported that they did not understand their surgical options after receiving an explanation from their healthcare provider

Participants Having Delayed or No Reconstruction Were Asked Whether Their Surgeon Clearly Explained Reconstruction Options Before Their Mastectomy:
- 83% ... Responded that they were well informed
- 17% ... Responded that they were not informed of reconstruction options

Chemotherapy Side Effects on Sexuality Patient Education:
- 87% ... Participants had **no** forewarning of the potential for sexual dysfunction from chemotherapy treatments
- 13% ... Participants had a pre-treatment discussion of potential side effects of chemotherapy treatment on future sexual function with a nurse or physician

Pre-Treatment Potential Sexual Dysfunction Discussion:
- 13% ... 1 minute
- 40% ... 2 – 4 minutes
- 7% .... 5 – 7 minutes
- 7% .... 8 – 10 minutes
- 13% ... 15 minutes
- 20% ... Over 15 minutes

Pre-Treatment Discussion Value:

Patients reported the value of the pre-treatment discussion at **6.4**.

Post Treatment Discussion About Potential Sexual Side Effects:

Participants were then asked if they had a discussion about sexual side effects after their chemotherapy treatments were completed. Only **5%** reported any healthcare provider discussing the potential impact. Therefore, between the two (pre- and post-treatment) discussions, a total of only **18%** of patients had a healthcare provider talk to them about the impact on sexuality anytime during or after treatment.

Length of Post-Treatment Discussion About Potential Sexual Dysfunction:

- **40%** ... 1 minute
- **0%** .... 2 – 4 minutes
- **20%** ... 5 – 7 minutes
- **20%** ... 8 – 10 minutes
- **0%** .... 15 minutes
- **20%** ... Over 15 minutes

Post-Treatment Discussion Value:

Patients rated the value of this post-treatment discussion at **3.5**. This finding indicates a discrepancy between what healthcare providers think a patient needs and what the patient finds valuable.

Participants were asked if they received any written information on sexuality issues in any of the material provided by healthcare workers before or after treatment:

- **29%** reported receiving some written information.
- The respondents rated the usefulness of this information at **5.6**

When asked if they questioned a physician/nurse about their sexual functioning during treatment:

- **32%** responded yes; however, **100%** reported having questions or problems.
- Those that asked questions about their sexual functioning rated the information provided by their healthcare providers a **4.1**, slightly less than somewhat helpful.
- When asked if a suggested intervention was effective, the respondents rated the intervention a **3.9**.

Participants were asked, *"How important do you think it is for a physician or nurse to discuss and offer suggestions about potential sexuality changes?"*:

- The group rated the need at a **9.4**.

When asked about providing written information about dealing with sexuality changes:

- They responded with a rating of **9.4**.

Focus Group Study

Post-Treatment Data

Resumption of Menstrual Period in Premenopausal Women Following Chemotherapy:

- 75% ... Did not resume periods; remained in menopausal state
- 18% ... Restarted their periods within the first five months after completion of treatment
- 7% .... Restarted their periods within the first year after completion of treatment

Post-Treatment Pregnancy:

- 3% .... Became Pregnant After Treatment

Patient Side Effects
Experienced One Year After Chemotherapy Treatment

Side Effect of Treatment	Percentage of Change From Time of Diagnosis to One Year After Treatment
Orgasm Ability	47% Decrease
Sex Drive	42% Decrease
Self Body Image	24% Decrease
Energy	22% Decrease
Painful Intercourse	163% Increase
Vaginal Dryness	158% Increase
Hot Flashes	83% Increase
Depression	75% Increase
Night Sweats	65% Increase
Insomnia	61% Increase
Anxiety	33% Increase
Mood Swings	22% Increase
Anger / Aggression	12% Increase
Weight Gain	54% Gained

Appendix C

Conclusion

Greatest Challenge

The final question asked the respondents to indicate their greatest present challenge from a pre-selected list by ranking each item in order of importance. As indicated in the chart below, the fear of recurrence was the number one greatest challenge of women in the focus groups.

- 56% ... Fear of recurrence
- 23% ... Side effects of treatment
- 8% ... Relationship
- 7% ..... Insurance
- 4% ..... Job lock*
- 2% ..... Social/career barriers

*Unable to change jobs because insurance benefits are tied to current employer.

What We Learned About Chemotherapy Treated Women:

- Sexuality side effects experienced during treatment were not limited to the treatment period.
- Many of the side effects that were thought to be treatment limited increased at one year post-treatment rather than decreased after treatment completion. Side effects that increased included: vaginal dryness, hot flashes and painful intercourse. Numerous other side effects of treatment failed to return to pre-treatment levels, which reduced over-all quality of life.
- Women often interpreted their sexual dysfunction as originating from personal lack of psychological strength to cope with their cancer diagnosis instead of being a side effect of treatment common to most women undergoing chemotherapy.
- Sexuality issues must be brought out of the medical treatment closet in order to address patients' needs.

BIBLIOGRAPHY

Bibliography

Chapter 1: Sexuality After Cancer Treatment
- (NWHRC) National Women's Health Resource Center, & (ARHP) Association of Reproductive Health Professionals. (n.d.). Women's Sexual Health: Provider Survey. Retrieved October 8, 2015, from http://www.arhp.org/publications-and-resources/studies-and-surveys/shy-survey
- Panjari, M., Bell, R., & Davis, S. (2011). Sexual Function after Breast Cancer. *The Journal of Sexual Medicine*, 8(1), 294-302. doi:10.1111/j.1743-6109.2010.02034.x
- Melisko, M., Goldman, M., & Rugo, H. (2010). Amelioration of Sexual Adverse Effects in the Early Breast Cancer Patient. *Journal of Cancer Survivorship*. doi:10.1007/s11764-010-0130-1
- Panjari, M., Bell, R., & Davis, S. (2011). Sexual Function after Breast Cancer. *The Journal of Sexual Medicine*, 8(1), 294-302. doi:10.1111/j.1743-6109.2010.02034.x

Chapter 5: Vaginal Dryness and Painful Intercourse
- Agarwal, A., Deepinder, F., Cocuzza, M., Short, R., & Evenson, D. (2008). Effect of vaginal lubricants on sperm motility and chromatin integrity: A prospective comparative study. *Fertility and Sterility*, 375-379.
- Chollet, J. (2011). Efficacy and safety of ultra-low-dose Vagifem (10 mcg). *Patient Preference and Adherence PPA*, 571-571. doi:10.2147/PPA.S22940
- Effective Treatments for Sexual Problems. (n.d.). Retrieved September 15, 2015, from http://www.menopause.org/for-women/sexual-health-menopause-online/effective-treatments-for-sexual-problems

Chapter 6: Urinary Changes
- Chollet, J. (2011). Efficacy and safety of ultra-low-dose Vagifem (10 mcg). *Patient Preference and Adherence PPA*, 571-571. doi:10.2147/PPA.S22940

Chapter 7: Hot Flashes and Night Sweats
- Clayton, A., Pradko, J., Croft, H., Montano, C., Leadbetter, R., Bolden-Watson, C., . . . Metz, A. (2002). Prevalence of Sexual Dysfunction Among Newer Antidepressants. *J. Clin. Psychiatry The Journal of Clinical Psychiatry*, 357-366.

Chapter 9: Sleep Problems
- What to Know About Hot Flashes, Hormone & Sleep. (2007). *National Sleep Foundation, 2007: Sleep in America*. doi:10.1016/j.sleh.2015.04.006

Bibliography

Chapter 10: Depression and Anxiety
- *Webster's New Collegiate Dictionary*. (1973). Springfield, Mass.: G. & C. Merriam.

Chapter 11: Value of Exercise
- Greenleaf, J., & Kozlowski, S. (1982). Physiological Consequences of Reduced Physical Activity During Bed Rest. *Exercise and Sport Sciences Reviews*, 84-119.
- Winningham, M. (2001). Strategies for Managing Cancer-Related Fatigue Syndrome. *American Cancer Society*, 92(4), 988-997. doi:10.1002/1097-0142(20010815)92:4 3.0.CO;2-O

Chapter 14: Drugs That Lower Your Sex Drive
- Breast Cancer Index. (n.d.). Retrieved October 8, 2015, from http://www.breastcancerindex.com
- *Physicians' Desk Reference* (58th ed.). (2004). Montvale, NJ: Thomson PDR.

Chapter 16: Increasing Female Sexual Pleasure
- Basson, R. (2011). The Female Sexual Response: A Different Model. *Journal of Sex & Marital Therapy*, 26(1), 51-65. doi:10.1080/009262300278641
- Clinical Fact Sheets: Female Sexual Response. (n.d.). Retrieved October 8, 2015, from http://www.arhp.org/publications-and-resources/clinical-fact-sheets/female-sexual-response

Chapter 17: Desire-Enhancing Medications and Supplements
- Ito, T., Polan, M., Whipple, B., & Trant, A. (2006). The Enhancement of Female Sexual Function with ArginMax, a Nutritional Supplement, Among Women Differing in Menopausal Status. *Journal of Sex & Marital Therapy*, 369-378. PMID: 16959660
- U.S. Food and Drug Administration. (2015, August 18). Retrieved October 8, 2015, from http://www.fda.gov/NewsEvents/Newsroom/PressAnnouncements/ucm458734.htm

Chapter 18: Reclaiming Your Life After Cancer
- Cloud, H., & Townsend, J. (1992). *Boundaries: When To Say Yes, When To Say No To Take Control of Your Life*. Grand Rapids, Mich.: Zondervan Pub. House.

Index

A

Addyi® ... 125
aggression ... 3, 187
alcohol ... 116
anatomy ... 21
anger ... 3, 187
anxiety ... 3, 81, 85, 187
   medications ... 87
   symptoms ... 84
ArginMax® ... 155
aromatase inhibitors (AIs) ... 101, 116
arousal ... 145
arousal time ... 141

B

body image ... 3, 13, 187
body massage ... 139
Breast Cancer Index (BCI) study ... 117
breast reconstruction procedures ... 173
   DIEP ... 174
   Fixed-volume Implant ... 173
   IGAP ... 176
   Latissimus Dorsi ... 175
   PAP ... 177
   SGAP ... 176
   TAP ... 175
   Tissue Expander ... 173
   TRAM ... 174
   TUG ... 177

C

capsular contracture ... 173
carbohydrates ... 104
cervix ... 26
clitoris ... 21, 199
clonidine ... 68
communication ... 144
cortisol ... 164
counseling ... 86
CPAP ... 79
cystitis ... 62

D

dating ... 112
depression ... 3, 81, 82, 187
   medications ... 87
   symptoms ... 83
desire ... 135
desire-enhancing medication ... 153

E

endorphins ... 94
energy ... 3, 187
Eros Therapy ... 146
estradiol ... 31
estriol ... 31
estrogen ... 31
estrone ... 31
exercise ... 93

Index

F
fatigue ... 12, 71
female sexual pathway ... 127
Female Sexual Response Cycle ... 142

G
gabapentin ... 68
Ginkgo biloba ... 156
Ginseng ... 156
Glycemic Index ... 105
G-Spot ... 25

H
hernia ... 174
hormones ... 12, 31
horny goat weed ... 156
hot flashes ... 3, 65, 187
   frequency ... 66
   medication ... 67
hypothyroidism ... 37

I
insomnia ... 3, 75, 95, 187
   medications ... 77
intercourse, painful ... 3, 43, 187

K
Kegel exercises ... 60, 61

L
labia majora ... 21, 199
labia minora ... 21, 199
L-arginine ... 155
lubrication ... 25
lymphatic system ... 95

M
mastectomy ... 14
medications ... 13, 86
menopause
   medically-induced ... 38
   natural ... 37
menstrual period ... 35
microsurgery ... 176
mood swings ... 3, 81, 187

N
nasal strips ... 79
night sweats ... 65
   frequency ... 66
   medication ... 67
nutrition ... 101

O
orgasm ... 3, 147, 187
oxytocin ... 128, 148

P
patient education ... 2
perimenopausal ... 34
postmenopausal ... 34
premenopausal ... 34
professional counseling ... 86
progesterone ... 31, 36
prolactin ... 128
psychiatrist ... 90
psychotherapy ... 86

Q
Quality of Life Assessment
   Post-Assessment ... 167
   Pre-Assessment ... 19

INDEX

R

reconstruction ... 15
recreational drugs ... 116
rest ... 93
romance ... 135

S

Scream Cream ... 157
sensual massage ... 139
seroma ... 174
sex drive ... 3, 11, 115, 123, 187
sex drive-reducing medications ... 115
sexual abuse ... 16
Sexuality After Breast Cancer Treatment focus group ... 2, 181
sexual side effects ... 7
sleep apnea ... 77
sleep problems ... 75
snoring ... 77
SNRIs (serotonin–norepinephrine reuptake inhibitors) ... 87
SSRIs (selective serotonin reuptake inhibitors) ... 87

T

tamoxifen ... 101, 116
testosterone ... 31, 35, 36, 154
thyroid gland ... 36
touch ... 137

U

urinary changes ... 59
urinary incontinence ... 59
    stress incontinence ... 60
    urge incontinence ... 60
urinary tract infection ... 62
urogynecologist ... 61
urologist ... 61
uterus ... 26

V

vagina ... 24
vaginal dilators ... 144, 179
vaginal dilator therapy ... 179
vaginal dryness ... 3, 43, 187
vaginal stenosis ... 179
Vitamin B complex ... 157
vulva ... 21

W

weight gain ... 3, 15, 101, 187
words ... 136

Y

Yohimbe ... 156

Z

Zestra® ... 156

Notes

Notes

TEAR-OUT SUPPLEMENT

A Message to the Sexual Partner

Your partner has undergone treatment for her cancer. The good news is that cancer treatment has increased cancer survival rates to an all-time high. The not-so-good news is that cancer treatment leaves behind lingering side effects that can impact a couple's sexual relationship. However, despite these sexual side effects, most partners and patients agree that they would not have chosen to forgo cancer treatment. The question after treatment ends is, *"What can we do to address these side effects and restore our sexual relationship to its fullest?"*

To address this issue, I have written this comprehensive guide to your partner describing why the side effects occurred and what steps of action she can take to address each of the side effects. In the next few pages, I am addressing you, her sexual partner, with tips to help her through this transition to restoring your sex life. As a sexual partner, you provide a pivotal role. The following information is a brief summary of how you can be most helpful. If you would like to understand more about what your partner faces, you may wish to read the rest of this book.

What Has Happened?
First, it is essential to understand that chemotherapy drugs greatly decrease hormones that control sexuality. The main hormones affected are estrogen and testosterone. Estrogen reduction causes vaginal dryness, lack of lubrication during foreplay, painful intercourse and numerous other side effects that impact sexuality. Testosterone reduction causes a decrease in: desire, genital and nipple sensitivity during foreplay, the ability to become sexually aroused and the ability to experience an orgasm. These side effects are caused by the impact of cancer treatment on her hormones, not because of her cancer. After cancer treatment, approximately 70 percent of women share these same sexual difficulties.

Sexuality After Cancer Treatment

What Can You Do?
It is extremely important to understand that sexual changes are not caused by her personal rejection of you as a partner. The next essential thing to know is that she needs your understanding, patience and support as she works to restore her sexuality. Losing her sexual desire and the ability to be an active sexual partner is difficult. She needs an understanding partner. Unlike many other side effects, you are the only person who can participate in her sexual healing.

What Do You Need To Know?
As a partner, you must have an accurate view of female sexuality. Regretfully, much of what is learned about sex is from the media—a man meets a woman and within a few minutes they become involved in a passionate encounter that brings screams of delight from the female. For a female, this becomes problematic; it is not reality, but sex made for TV. This is NOT how female sexuality functions.

Women are completely different than men when it comes to sexual arousal. Men are driven by the hormone testosterone and can be stimulated quickly. Women are driven by a complex mixture of mental, relational and self-esteem issues that makes arousal more complicated and takes longer. Understanding the differences in arousal time is essential.

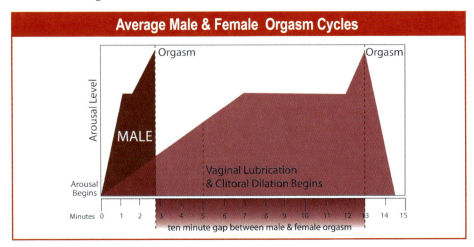

Men are like a microwave and women are like a crock-pot.
Rule #1: Women need lots of foreplay to be sexually ready. Slow down!

A Message to the Sexual Partner

Jerry Seinfeld said it best: *"Seems to me the basic conflict between men and women, sexually, is that men are like **firemen**. To men, sex is an emergency, and no matter what we're doing we can be ready in two minutes. Women, on the other hand, are like **fire**. They're exciting, but the conditions have to be exactly right for it to occur."* How true.

The next thing you need to understand is the female genital anatomy.

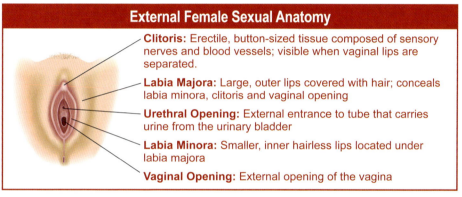

External Female Sexual Anatomy

Clitoris: Erectile, button-sized tissue composed of sensory nerves and blood vessels; visible when vaginal lips are separated.

Labia Majora: Large, outer lips covered with hair; conceals labia minora, clitoris and vaginal opening

Urethral Opening: External entrance to tube that carries urine from the urinary bladder

Labia Minora: Smaller, inner hairless lips located under labia majora

Vaginal Opening: External opening of the vagina

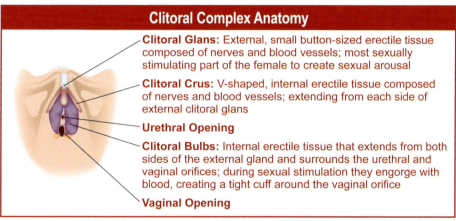

Clitoral Complex Anatomy

Clitoral Glans: External, small button-sized erectile tissue composed of nerves and blood vessels; most sexually stimulating part of the female to create sexual arousal

Clitoral Crus: V-shaped, internal erectile tissue composed of nerves and blood vessels; extending from each side of external clitoral glans

Urethral Opening

Clitoral Bulbs: Internal erectile tissue that extends from both sides of the external gland and surrounds the urethral and vaginal orifices; during sexual stimulation they engorge with blood, creating a tight cuff around the vaginal orifice

Vaginal Opening

The clitoris is the erectile portion of the female genitals that is equivalent to the male penis. The female clitoris and the male penis originate from the same hormonally sensitive tissues while a fetus is in the uterus.

For a female, the clitoris contains the most sexually sensitive tissues in her body. The clitoris has approximately 8,000 nerves and a network of erectile tissue like the penis. Only a small portion of the clitoris is visible; the majority is hidden under the skin.

Sexuality After Cancer Treatment

When a woman is accepting of touch from a sexual partner, messages are sent to the brain through the spinal column that set off a number of physical changes—blood flow increases to the vulva, clitoris, vagina and breasts, which causes the tissues to engorge with blood and increase in size. The vaginal wall secretes a slippery fluid for lubrication that causes an aroused woman to feel wet. Heart and respiration rates increase. Engorgement causes the covering over the external clitoris to retract, exposing an erect clitoris. The internal clitoral legs and bulbs from a tight cuff around the vagina from the filling of blood which causes engorgement. The nipples become erect. These are signals of sexual readiness.

After chemotherapy, this arousal process is slowed down. But, only when this readiness process has occurred is penetration comfortable. Because of this, you must plan to enhance your efforts to increase her arousal potential. This is where your understanding and cooperation are key to helping her restore her sexual function.

What Does She Need?
First on the agenda is relationship. Foreplay for a woman is based on how you relate to her as a person. The words you say to her that confirm her value and attractiveness as a sexual partner are essential. Your participation in her life through conversation, awareness of her presence and support with challenges all prime her sexual pump. Taking the trash out or helping with the dishes is often the first step in foreplay for a woman. If you want better and more frequent sex, spend more time on your relationship with her. Results are guaranteed.

Physical fatigue is also a saboteur of sex. Plan to help her save energy for sex by offering to help around the house or by hiring someone to help with household chores when her energy is low.

Plan a date night. Women look forward to a special time, activity or a meal out. Take the opportunity during this time to verbalize her value to you as a partner.

She needs WORDS, WORDS, WORDS. A woman derives so much of her sexual self-esteem from what you say to her. Tell her about her sexual attractiveness to you. Compliment her. Write notes of love to her. Praise her in front of other people. Remember, words are like money, she can never have too much.

A Message to the Sexual Partner

How Do You Plan For A Sexual Encounter?
When planning for a sexual encounter, it is essential that a woman feels safe from interruptions. You can help by putting a lock on the bedroom door or sending children to a friend's house.

Plan ahead by purchasing a massage oil (natural oils are best) and a sexual lubricant. Because vaginal dryness is a problem caused by her lack of vaginal lubrication, a lubricant is required to avoid friction and discomfort.

What Are Her Sexual Arousal Zones?
- **Mouth, Lips, Ears, Neck and Buttocks:** These areas are all sensitive to sexually stimulating touch.
- **Breast and Nipples:** These are very sexually stimulating areas for most women. However, save them until you have stimulated the other sensitive areas listed above (leave genitals for last).
- **Clitoris:** The most erogenous zone in the female body. The internal portion, which lies under the skin for about four inches on each side of the visible portion, responds to light pressure. Pressure stimulates the clitoral legs and bulbs to fill with blood. The external, button-sized portion is usually too sensitive for direct touch until a woman is fully aroused. Gentle pressure around the external clitoris is preferred by most women.

What Do the Experts Say?
Dr. Rosemary Basson, a specialist in sexuality, recommends that women who have low desire submit to their partner's sexual stimulation and, after adequate simulation, desire will come. This technique has proven very successful for many cancer-treated patients. She also recommends sensual massage as a tool to create desire. This technique requires a dedicated partner who understands that previous sexual techniques may need to change after treatment. There is now a need for prolonged foreplay to create sexual desire. These changes, however, can serve to bring a new joy to the sexual relationship and bring the two of you closer as a couple.

Sexuality After Cancer Treatment

How You Can "Turn Her Back On"

If letter grades were given to sexually arousing stimulation, sensual massage would score an "A" rating by most women. Sensual body massage given by you prior to sexual intercourse is a guaranteed pleasure stimulator. During the massage, stimulating all the erogenous zones previously listed creates heightened sexual arousal.

The guiding rule is slow, tender touch. Don't rush! Sensual massage is extremely helpful for women who have lowered desire due to cancer treatment. It allows a woman to relax and be slowly stimulated to arousal.

Sensual Body Massage Tips:

- Select a location for the massage. A hard surface, massage table or bed work well.
- Be sure that the temperature in the room is warm.
- Protect the bed or massage surface with a sheet or towel.
- Turn down the lights, light candles and turn on soft music.
- Use a towel or sheet to cover the body. Keep the body covered during the massage. Only uncover the body part you are massaging while keeping the rest of the body covered.
- Make sure the body is positioned straight on the massage surface to relieve stress and release pressure.
- Warm your hands and the massage oil if needed. Apply the oil to your warm hands and not directly to the skin.
- Begin the massage with the face down. Use gentle stroking or circular motions on her back. Do not use heavy, deep or excessive pressure. Massage the muscles and not the bones, especially near the spine. Now move to the more sensitive zone and touch, lick or kiss them.
- Get feedback; ask if the pressure is too deep or if the temperature of the room is comfortable. When moving to another part of the body, ask if massage in this area is pleasurable. During the massage, pay attention to her body tension and relaxation. Relaxed muscle tension, sighing or quiet moaning with pleasure are all signs that the massage is successful. Communication and chemistry between the two of you will make this a success.
- The buttocks are very sensual and respond when a kneading motion is used because of the large amount of soft tissue in the buttocks. Kneading

A Message to the Sexual Partner

is similar to the way a baker kneads bread. The motion is very simple. First, press the palms down on the muscle tissue; then, push your fingers together into the tissue and move the tissue upward in a lifting motion. Relax the tension of the hands and repeat.

- After the back of the body is fully massaged, the front of the body is massaged while lying face up. Stroke the thighs allowing the stroke to come near the genitals, without directly touching them. Next, move to the chest area.
- Massage the chest area around the breast while leaving the breast tissue for last. After massaging the chest around the breast, start to massage the breasts using gentle pressure around the nipples but avoid massaging the nipples. Nipple erection is a sign of sexual stimulation. When a high level of sexual stimulation occurs, the nipples will reflect the arousal by becoming extremely erect. At the same time, you will notice that body tension noticeably increases, and the pectoralis muscles tighten causing the breast mound to rise as your strokes come near the nipple. Allow this sexual tension to build by continuing to come close to the nipples without touching them. When sexual tension is high, the nipples respond best to very gentle pressure of licking.
- Genital touch is reserved until last. Apply generous amounts of vaginal lubricant to your fingers and use a very light, gentle touch to the external area of the vulva. Move gradually into the folds of the labia. As swelling occurs, begin softly stroking the sides of the clitoris without touching or applying pressure to the clitoris. Many women find direct pressure to the clitoris early in arousal to be uncomfortable.
- As vaginal congestion increases, attempt to enter the vagina with a lubricated finger. If the vaginal entry is tight, continue external stimulation to increase arousal and then gently reattempt to enter a finger into the vagina. If penetration is attempted and is painful, stop. If you find you must stop, verbalize your understanding and explain that you want to continue to bring her pleasure even if penetration is not possible. Sexual arousal, even without intercourse, increases the blood flow to the genitals and vagina, causing healing of the tissues. Repeated arousal is helpful to restore her sexuality.

Women love the closeness and attention that massage brings to the relationship. Massage causes a woman to feel special. Sensual massage

Sexuality After Cancer Treatment

allows a hormone-deficient woman the time and stimulation needed to reach the sexual excitement stage.

Incorporating sensual massage extends the time of foreplay for the cancer-treated woman while her partner stimulates all her erogenous tissues. When the massaging partner does not receive reciprocal stimulation during the massage, this delays their sexual arousal. This delay allows the female partner to reach a high level of arousal before penetration is attempted. The full sexual readiness of the female partner before penetration decreases the potential of sexual discomfort or pain. Sensual massage becomes the key to both partners experiencing a satisfying sexual experience.

Remember:
- Her level of sex hormones determines how quickly she can become aroused. Because cancer-treated women are prone to low sex hormone levels, arousal may require an extended time for foreplay for arousal to occur. Slow and steady sensual touching is one of the best ways to create sexual arousal.
- Never touch her external or internal genitals without lubrication or wet fingers. These tissues are dry from cancer treatment and are easily irritated. Ask if you can apply the lubricant to her external genital tissues and then to her vagina. Make this an exciting part of foreplay. Apply the lubricant with a very slow and gentle touch. Don't hurry. Women don't respond well to a fast hand!

How You Become Her Hero
Restoring your sexual life after your partner's cancer treatment is an intimate partnership. A partnership where you are pivotal to her success. You can become her chief encourager to work through the sexual challenges she faces after cancer treatment. Often, women feel that their partners don't find them as desirable because of the physical changes they have undergone during treatment and their lack of sex drive. Your words and your attention can help change that perception. You can become a joyful, willing participant in helping her restore her sexual desire and arousal. You are the key to her sexual healing and helping her find joy in sex again. You can become her hero.